Organ Transplants:
A Patient's Guide

Organ Transplants

A Patient's Guide

The Massachusetts General Hospital
Organ Transplant Team
and H. F. Pizer

Harvard University Press
Cambridge, Massachusetts
London, England
1991

Copyright © 1991 by H. F. Pizer
All rights reserved
Printed in the United States of America
10 9 8 7 6 5 4 3 2 1

This book is printed on acid-free paper, and its binding
materials have been chosen for strength and durability.

Library of Congress Cataloging-in-Publication Data

Organ transplants : a patient's guide / the Massachusetts
   General Hospital Organ Transplant Team and
   H. F. Pizer.
      p.   cm.
   Includes index.
   ISBN 0-674-64235-X (alk. paper)
   1. Transplantation of organs, tissues, etc.—Popular
   works.
2. Patient education.   I. Pizer, Hank.
II. Massachusetts General Hospital. Organ
Transplant Team.
   [DNLM: 1. Organ Procurement—popular works.
2. Organ Transplantation—popular works.
WO 660 0687]
RD120.75.074   1991
617.9'5—dc20
DNLM/DLC
for Library of Congress   91-7083
                                                      CIP

Designed by Gwen Frankfeldt

For all organ donors and transplant patients,
past, present, and future

Contents

Preface

The first organ transplanted at the MGH was a kidney, and the operation took place on February 27, 1963. The recipient, a young man in his twenties, was suffering from severe kidney destruction due to glomerulonephritis, one of the many auto-immune disorders in which the body's immune system acts destructively against its own tissues and organs. The kidney he received was donated by one of his parents.

In the early 1960s organ transplantation was still almost unknown to the general public, and was considered something of a curiosity even by physicians. While it had been known for some time that transplant rejection could be controlled to a considerable degree by the administration of X-rays, the very early transplants of the mid-1950s had been accomplished without any special measures to control rejection, and with only limited success. Later on, a few operations were performed after administering moderate to large doses of whole-body irradiation to suppress normal immune function. Although this did succeed in blunting the immune response to transplanted kidneys, it did so in quite an uncertain way, and was accompanied by many undesirable side-effects.

Meanwhile, laboratory research was demonstrating that certain chemical agents—especially cortisone-like drugs—could be quite effective for a period of time in delaying the

vigorous inflammatory response that causes transplant rejection. And, in 1962, another considerable step forward was
made when azathioprine (Imuran) became available to inhibit
rejection. Other than the cortisone-like compounds, azathioprine was the first truly effective chemical immunosuppressive
to become available. Its side-effects, mainly in suppressing
bone marrow function, were significant, but quite manageable.
With these new tools to control immune rejection available,
the time seemed right for the MGH to enter the field of human
transplantation.

There are three major hurdles standing in the way of successfully transplanting any organ. First, one must have a suitable technique for placing the new organ into the recipient's
body in such a way that it will function promptly and effectively. Herein lie the formidable technical difficulties faced by
the surgeons when performing a transplant. Second, one must
be able to control the powerful and persistent immune response to foreign tissues and cells—the rejection reaction. And
third, there is the problem of organ availability. An appropriate
organ must be identified, removed from its donor, maintained
in a viable state, and delivered at the right time to the recipient's hospital.

The surgical problems of transplantation clearly differ from
one organ to another. Although they are by no means trivial,
before the first transplant was attempted the foundations for
solving these problems were already well laid from prior experience in performing a wide array of other operations. In
the case of the kidney, for example, the necessary methods for
joining blood vessels and reconstructing the urinary tract had
already been quite amply perfected; although the technique
currently employed has undergone a number of valuable re-
finements, by and large it was described and performed in the
1950s by René Küss, a French surgeon. Similarly, successful
techniques for transplanting the liver, heart, lungs, and pancreas have been based on the earlier efforts of surgeons who
were not replacing old organs with new ones. Indeed, transplant surgeons have benefited enormously from the great ac-

complishments of colleagues working in other areas of surgery. The result has been the refinement of surgical techniques to solve extraordinarily difficult problems, along with striking improvement in outcome for modern transplant recipients.

The control of transplant rejection has been an interesting and complex story. When we began our program at MGH, there were perhaps half a dozen institutions in the United States, and a very few others in other countries, in which there was any serious interest in the fundamental biology of tissue transplantation. As the intrinsic interest of the field became evident to scientists—and its practical importance more and more pressing because surgeons were increasingly performing transplant operations—the discipline of transplantation biology grew rapidly. In a very short time, the effort to find new ways of selectively inhibiting the immune system grew from a cottage industry into a major activity. A large number of able investigators began to work in the rapidly advancing field of immunogenetics, which is concerned with the relationship between the genetic makeup and the immune response. Progress was made, for example, in tissue typing to test compatibility between donor and recipient, and in the use of biological agents such as antibodies to prevent or treat acute organ rejection. Transplant rejection continues, however, to be a supremely important issue. Even though newer agents, including cyclosporine and others, have improved our ability to control rejection, the requirement for continuing treatment with immunosuppressing medications that have troublesome side-effects leaves much room for further progress.

By the mid-1960s, a small number of kidney transplants were being performed in Boston at both the Peter Bent Brigham (now the Brigham and Women's) Hospital and the MGH. In those days, most of the donors were family members who had been very carefully screened on the basis of their health status, motivation, and their understanding of the risks and benefits involved in giving a vital organ. For quite a while the possibility of using a deceased patient as a donor was felt to be thoroughly impractical. There was a widespread belief in the field that it would be impossible to remove an organ from a dead patient and get it into a working position in a recipient before it had suffered irreversible damage from lack of circulation. In those days society had not yet accepted the concept of brain death—of declaring a patient dead when the brain ceased to function—so no thought of removing an organ from a donor could be entertained until all evidence of heart action had ceased.

As we began to explore the use of deceased donors, it gradually became clear that we would have to consider donors in other hospitals, and that a new interdependence between institutions would have to develop. I spoke with Drs. Joseph Murray and Francis Moore of the Peter Bent Brigham Hospital about the possibility of establishing a cooperative exchange system among Boston hospitals for this purpose. This seemed all the more reasonable after one notable experience I had with Dr. Moore. One Sunday morning, he called me at home to say that he had read in the newspaper of a policeman in our intensive care unit at the MGH who had been shot in the head while trying to stop a robbery. At this time, Dr. Moore was in the early stages of his effort to transplant the liver, working primarily with laboratory dogs. However, he had encountered a patient whom he thought he might be able to help with a new liver. Time was short for this person. A new organ had to be found very urgently, or the patient would die. I agreed to go immediately to the MGH to look into the possibility of securing the liver from the brain-dead policeman, should he prove to be a suitable donor. I well remember the circumstances. The man's wife was courageous and generous. The events followed in rapid order. We removed the dead policeman's liver, and under sterile conditions and at low temperature, sped it across town to the Brigham Hospital, where Dr. Moore performed the first liver transplant in the region.

After that, we became even more serious about setting up an organization for organ exchange. That effort culminated in the establishment of the Boston Inter-hospital Organ Bank. With our colleagues at the several Boston hospitals that by that time also had entered the field of organ transplantation, we set up a system of charges, and a system for organ distribution, which was one of the first in the world to address these complicated issues. Later, as additional hospitals entered the field, we expanded the organization to include the entire New England region. This organization became the New England Organ Bank, with a staff of many employees, vehicles to transport organs from one institution to another, a modern tissue typing laboratory, and an extensive structure of committees to provide for its various functions. Now that organs can be successfully transported over fairly large distances, and there are, of course, many more organs that can be transplanted, the work of the Organ Bank has increased enormously. As is described in Chapter 1, we now have a nationwide organization for organ sharing.

In a relatively short time kidney transplantation began to feel almost routine, and we began to look into other areas of transplantation. The heart seemed the logical next organ. Lively formal discussion took place on two different occasions, first in 1974 and again in 1979, to evaluate the possibility of establishing a heart transplant program at our hospital. On both occasions, it was finally decided not to proceed with this then experimental and very expensive treatment. In those days, heart transplantation was of uncertain value for the recipient, although it was already known at that time that the results in certain patients could be excellent and long lasting. However, after advances in the management of rejection reactions, along with other technical improvements, the expense began to decline, and heart transplantation was at last begun at the MGH in November 1985. As you will see in Chapter 7 and in the words of the heart recipients in Chapter 10, this is now a highly successful and rewarding endeavor.

When our plan to proceed in heart transplantation was delayed, we turned out attention to another organ, the liver. In the early 1980s, with the introduction of cyclosporine, the results with liver replacement had begun to improve quite dramatically. On May 21, 1983, we initiated the first liver transplant program in New England with an operation on a young woman suffering from terminal cirrhosis caused by a viral infection. The program has steadily grown and prospered with much success in improving the lot of the very sick patients who come to our group for this treatment of last resort.

Our next step was to explore transplanting the pancreas for the treatment of advanced diabetes. Here, we elected to treat patients suffering from both advanced diabetes and kidney failure as a consequence of it. Our first combined kidney and pancreas transplant was performed on April 3, 1986, and it was another New England first. Again, experience with the care of these severely ill patients has helped us to understand better the disease they face, and to concentrate on plans for further improving their lot. With the realization that a successful pancreas transplant is currently the only known cure for the metabolic complications of diabetes (such as kidney failure, blindness, and cardiovascular disease), this approach cries out for further improvement and application.

Much remains to be done in the field of organ transplantation. The shortage of donor organs continues to limit the number of desperately ill patients who can be treated with transplants; it is vital to develop better means of securing and distributing donor organs. Meanwhile, we will also continue to explore other alternatives. The possibilities now under consideration include mechanical devices for some organs, such as the heart, and organs from animals that have acceptable physiological and immunological characteristics. Future advances in the field of immunology will lead to more effective ways of controlling organ rejection. One long-standing goal is to be able to establish a persistent state of tolerance to the transplant, so that after the initial treatment no further immunosuppressive medication would be necessary. There would be no drug side-effects and many fewer late complications. Should this become possible, it would be feasible to transplant many other organs and tissues besides the life-sustaining ones we currently replace. Beyond this lies a host of other fascinating possibilities. Needed organs and tissues might be fashioned in the laboratory, started from only a few "seed" cells. After all, the human embryo develops from just one fertilized cell, which bears the full genetic complement. The use of large sheets of skin cells formed in tissue culture from small bits of the patient's own skin already affords an example of how the body's own cells can be used to create a needed tissue, in this case for the treatment of extensive burns. Some day we may even be able to transplant not only whole organs but minute functioning genes to overcome certain types of deficiencies, such as the lack of a normal source of insulin in diabetics.

From its beginning, transplantation presented society with difficult ethical and policy problems. Some have been resolved, while others remain. As future progress is made, new challenges of this sort will almost certainly arise. There can be no question, however, when one of our early transplant recipients strides into my office with a healthy smile on his face twenty-five years after his operation, that the effort has not only been exciting and fascinating, but also rewarding in the deepest human sense.

Paul Russell, M.D.
Former Chief, Transplantation Unit
Massachusetts General Hospital

Organ Transplants:
A Patient's Guide

Authors' Note

This book represents the views and medical opinions of the Massachusetts General Hospital Transplantation Service and, therefore, may differ somewhat in certain aspects from the approach at other transplant centers. Many different approaches to a given problem are equally acceptable, and many areas of medicine, including transplantation, are practiced differently at various institutions.

Although this text focuses on the MGH program, it should not be interpreted as suggesting that this institution has been any more than simply representative of what was happening in a number of other teaching centers more or less at the same time.

Further, this work is not intended to replace your own physician or transplant team, with whom you should consult before taking any medication, considering any change in medical treatment, or otherwise making a decision regarding your medical care.

1

The Donor Organ Network

On July 14, 1985, backstage at the Live Aid concert in Philadelphia, the Pennsylvania State Police asked the comedian Chevy Chase to go onstage and interrupt the concert. He was to tell a member of the audience, Stephen Flint, to report to the first aid station beneath the stadium.

Anxiously, Stephen made his way to the aid station, wondering if there was a family emergency. When he got there the medic told him reassuringly, "Stephen, the Transplantation Unit at the hospital called. They have a kidney for you." The moment Stephen had been waiting for had arrived. The medics made arrangements for the State Police to rush Stephen to the airport, where he took the next plane to Boston. By that evening he had his new kidney.

While most organ recipients are not called to surgery from an international rock concert, Stephen Flint's story illustrates the working of the sophisticated network that has developed in the past decade. This independent, national network of hospitals throughout North America, known as the United Network for Organ Sharing (UNOS), provides organs and tissues to nearly 15,000 recipients each year. Acknowledging that human organs are a vital national resource donated voluntarily in the spirit of altruism, this modern organ banking system— now supported by the U.S. government—distributes this "gift of life" without regard to the recipients' race, sex, ethnic background, or ability to pay. Without any element of commercialization, agencies that provide organs are designated as "OPA"—for organ procurement agency—only when they meet special standards that maximize the likelihood of successfully transplanting human organs. As of the beginning of 1990, there were seventy-two such OPAs in the United States.

Finding a Donor

The general method by which a donor kidney was found for Stephen Flint is now rather routine. Most often, a young person is in an automobile accident and suffers irreparable brain damage, called brain death. While the concept of brain death is now well accepted by both the medical and legal professions, it is a relatively new one in medical history.

The criteria for brain death were first presented in 1968, following a Harvard Medical School conference of experts in the fields of medicine, law, ethics, and the social sciences. Later, a Presidential Commission of similar authorities refined and clarified the guidelines. The Commission focused on two principal elements of the definition: an absence of all brain function and the irreversibility of the brain injury. Doctors assess brain function not only by evaluating the cerebrum (the portion of the brain that registers sensation, controls voluntary muscles, and coordinates mental processes) but also by evaluating the brain stem (which connects the cerebrum to the spinal cord, and which controls breathing and other vital functions). A brain-dead person is unable to take a breath without the assistance of a respirator (also called a ventilator), a machine that mechanically controls breathing. To confirm the absence of brain stem function, the potential donor is removed from the ventilator for a period of time long enough (usually one to two minutes) to raise the carbon dioxide content of the blood to the level that normally triggers a breath. If the person does not breathe, the respirator is replaced, and the confirmation of a functionless brain stem is made. Tracings of brain activity by electroencephalogram (EEG) also help make the assessment. Brain death should not be confused with prolonged coma, the so-called vegetative state. In unusual circumstances, such as the tragic case of Karen Anne Quinlan, a person may be deeply comatose, but not dead. In this situation, the patient retains brain stem function and breathes without mechanical assistance.

For many people—including many physicians—the concept of brain death is a challenge to basic emotions and beliefs. However, as a result of public and professional education, over the years we have come a long way in thinking of death as an absence of brain function. Loss of a person's pulse or breath may only be a sign of lost brain activity, and survival is possible for many minutes after cardiac arrest. For instance, provided resuscitation efforts are successful, the heart can stop for up to about five minutes without brain death. Or it can be removed from the body for a longer period during a heart transplant without damaging the brain. But each year perhaps twenty thousand relatively young and healthy people suffer brain death, dying prematurely from accidents, stroke, or brain tumors. With the determination of brain death, their otherwise healthy organs and tissues can be used for others.

Once Stephen Flint's donor was pronounced dead, the physician caring for the patient was obligated ethically to request permission from the family to donate the deceased person's organs. Recently, this obligation has been the subject of state legislation intended to increase awareness about organ donation. Many states, including Massachusetts, have so-called required request laws, which require physicians to discuss organ donation with a patient's relatives when suitable criteria apply. Although it was thought that these laws would increase the frequency of organ donation, so far "required request" has not proved to be beneficial in this regard.

At the time of renewing his (or her) driver's license, Stephen Flint's donor had indicated the desire to be an organ donor. Nevertheless, family permission was still obtained. Once this was granted, the donor's hospital contacted the local organ bank. A member of the organ bank staff rushed to the potential donor's bedside to assess whether this particular brain-dead patient was an acceptable candidate for organ and/ or tissue donation. First, age was considered. People older than sixty-five are generally not acceptable donors. A careful medical and social history was then obtained regarding the donor's past sexual and drug practices, either of which could have precluded giving an organ. Despite a satisfactory history, which indicated a low risk for disease, the donor's blood was sampled for exposure to hepatitis and AIDS. This is now standard practice. Other important medical factors were considered as well, and tests were run to assess the function of various organ systems. Since the donor's death was due to an unnatural cause—an automobile accident—the local Medical Examiner was contacted to sanction removing the organ(s). With these details completed, and with permission from the family and the attending physician, the OPA coordinator then assumed responsibility for managing the intravenous fluids of this declared-dead patient. The next task was to schedule the operations that would permit procuring the eyes, heart, liver, and kidneys. (Because of long bone fractures sustained in the accident, the patient was unable to donate bones.) The coordinator's next responsibility was to determine the potential recipients for each of these organs. One would be Stephen Flint.

That was the summer of 1985, and by then the coordinator had access to a relatively new computer-generated list of potential recipients living within the geographic region served by the organ bank. Today a nationwide computer list is available for identifying recipients. This breakthrough was the result of a 1983 public appeal by President Reagan for Jamie Fiske, an infant suffering from liver failure. In response to Jamie's need—and the needs of others like her—Congress held hearings to determine ways to maximize the availability of organs for transplantation. This effort culminated in the National Organ Transplant Act of 1984, which provided funding for a nationwide organ-sharing system, the Organ Procurement and Transplantation Network (OPTN). In 1986, the Department of Health and Human Services awarded the first contract to UNOS, thereby establishing the private, nonprofit network we have today.

Governed by a board of directors composed of transplant professionals, recipients, family members, and public representatives from ethics, medicine, law, religion, and health care financing, UNOS allocates organs to more than 250 transplant centers throughout the United States. With more than 20,000 people in the country awaiting the gift of life on any given day, a fundamental goal of UNOS is to ensure equity in the system. Recognizing the potential for commercial abuse, the National Transplant Act of 1984 prohibits the *sale* of organs. The goal of the system is to ensure that each organ that becomes available is transplanted in the most equitable and successful manner possible. The length of time a candidate has been on the UNOS waiting list is an essential determinant. However, other criteria, such as blood type, body size, and genetic match are also considered in selecting a recipient. These subjects are discussed in greater detail later in this book.

Unfortunately, only about four thousand donors are identified each year—obviously far fewer than the number needed to help all the seriously ill patients who might benefit from organ replacement. Moreover, according to statistics prepared by UNOS, the number of cadaveric (deceased) donors actually declined slightly from 1988 to 1989. There appear to be a number of reasons for the continuing shortfall. First, an organ remains viable for transplantation for only a very limited time following the determination of death. Second, some medical professionals are still reluctant to request permission from a grieving family. Third, more public education is needed to help families make the decision to donate.

On the evening of July 13, 1985, the family of the crash victim granted permission for organ donation, and the

OPA staff immediately looked for potential recipients. Candidates were selected based upon their time on the waiting list, medical urgency, and blood type, and, for organs other than the kidney, their compatibility for a proper size match with the replacement organ. The staff first looked for potential recipients living in the surrounding cities and state. (Today, with UNOS's national list and the ability to send kidneys long distances, a kidney recipient may be found living thousands of miles away.) When no appropriate person was found in the vicinity, the search was widened.

Next, tissue typing was performed to determine the best match for each kidney. (The kidney is the only organ for which the tissue match is a determining factor.) Samples of the donor's lymph nodes, which contain lymphocytes, a type of white blood cell valuable for the matching, were sent to the laboratory for analysis. Based on markers called antigens, these cells were then typed, and Stephen Flint was identified as a good prospect for receiving one of the kidneys. It was now time to find Stephen—and there was no time to waste.

The next step in the transplant process is to contact the surgeons who will be responsible for procuring each of the donor organs. They may have to travel to the donor hospital from three or four different medical institutions. For instance, one team might come from Boston to remove the heart, another from Chicago to retrieve the liver, a third group from New Haven for the pancreas, and a fourth from the donor hospital itself might obtain the kidneys. Arrangements for transporting each surgical team are made through the organ procurement agency. Helicopters and private jets, as well as ambulances, are used for utmost speed. Today, as many more surgeons have become proficient in organ procurement, local teams often conduct donor surgery, and less traveling is required.

The operations must be finely orchestrated. First, the heart transplant team divides the breastbone to expose the heart and major blood vessels, which are then visually inspected to see if the heart will be satisfactory for transplantation. Next, the liver team opens the abdomen and carefully dissects the blood vessels that supply the liver and intestines and the common bile duct that drains bile from the liver. The liver is then freed from its attachment to the diaphragm, leaving it suspended only by a large blood vessel, the inferior vena cava. Now, the pancreas team divides the "tail" of the pancreas from the nearby spleen, and then frees it from the surrounding donut of intestine, the duodenum. A portion of the duodenum is left attached to the pancreas for transplantation into the recipient. Finally, the kidney team prepares each kidney, with its ureteral tube, which transports urine from the kidney to the bladder. Now it is time to interrupt the blood supply to the donor organs. First, however, the organs must be quickly chilled and preserved in a special fluid, so they will withstand transit outside the body.

The transplant surgeons now arrest the heart with a potassium-containing solution, and swiftly, but carefully, remove it from the chest. Next the liver is removed, followed by the kidneys with their ureters. Finally, the pancreas, with its segment of duodenum, is freed. The reason for this sequence is to avoid contaminating the heart, liver, or kidneys with bacteria from the intestine, which may be present when the duodenum is dissected. After each organ is removed, it is bathed in ice-cold preservative fluid, placed in a cooler containing ice, and rushed off to the waiting transport. The entire donation process usually takes three or four hours.

Time is severely restricted for the surgical teams. The heart must be transplanted within four to six hours, so the team at the recipient's hospital generally begin their cardiac operation at the same time that the donor heart is being removed. The two groups maintain close contact by speaker telephones connecting the two remote operating suites. Until recently, such speed was necessary for liver replacement, as well. However, an improved preserving fluid developed by researchers at the University of Wisconsin now allows the liver to remain viable outside the body for up to twenty-four hours. Because the islets of Langerhans—the insulin-producing cells in the pancreas—are very sensitive to the absence of blood circulation, generally the pancreas must be transplanted within approximately six hours. The kidneys, once they are connected to a machine that delivers pulses of preserving solution, can be preserved up to seventy-two hours. And so there was ample time to contact Stephen Flint's family, track him down at the rock concert in Philadelphia, and get him back to Boston for his operation.

One final point—the American Council of Transplantation estimates that only about 15 percent of potential donors actually make the gift of life. As you read the stories of recipients whose lives have benefited from transplantation, keep in mind ways in which you might encourage and educate others in your community about the importance of organ donation. Donated organs are a most precious natural resource; and there is still much more to be done to make them available to people in need.

2

The Immune Barrier

"Millions of people have enjoyed their drama. This was the first time, I think, that a wholly unknown patient became the hero of headlines. Who knows whether it was the spectacle of mother love or the longing of the human race for eternal life that made these millions hope for the miracle of a supply of spare parts for human organs? The experiment has failed. It has shown that even the close kinship of mother and son is not sufficient to prevent rejection of an organ."

This letter, written on March 14, 1953, by Dr. Paul Benoist, recounts a tragic but historic event that caught the attention of ordinary people throughout France. The patient was sixteen-year-old Marius Renard, who on Christmas Day entered medical history by receiving a kidney transplanted from his mother.

In December 1952, young Marius, a carpenter's assistant living outside Paris, was severely injured in a fall from the fourth floor of a construction site. Rushed to a nearby hospital, he was dispatched to surgery. His pelvis was opened, revealing a badly injured right kidney. Assuming the presence of a normal left kidney, the attending surgeon removed the damaged one. Days passed, and Marius failed to make urine. His condition wors-

ened. He was transferred by ambulance to a hospital in
Paris.

At the receiving hospital, doctors soon discovered that
Marius Renard had been born without a left kidney. Unless something could be done—and done soon—the boy
would lapse into coma and die. His mother, Gilberte Renard, had read a newspaper story about a child who reportedly had been saved by a kidney transplanted from
his mother. Gilberte begged for an operation. Skeptical of
the newspaper account, the doctors warned that a transplant would not succeed: her kidney would be rejected
by her son's immune system. But Gilberte insisted. Without the operation her son would die. What would any
mother do in such a case? Their blood types were compatible. The doctors had to try.

And so on Christmas Day, mother and son were simultaneously wheeled into the operating room. Two
teams of surgeons labored in tandem. Gilberte's left kidney was removed, and in less than an hour was attached
to her son's blood supply. Immediately, the replacement
kidney began to produce urine, cleansing Marius of the
waste products that were killing him. The French press
heard of the operation and began reporting on the patient's recovery with both hope and joy. It appeared to be
a Christmas miracle.

But on New Year's Day Marius began to have pain.
Still there was hope, as his mother's kidney continued to
function. By the fourth of January, however, his temperature rose. There was an infection. But the kidney was still
working. At two weeks past surgery, the kidney was still
producing urine. Finally, by the third week after transplantation, the kidney failed. The boy's body filled with
toxic waste products. He could not eat. His energy
sagged. Despite all medical efforts he was lapsing into
coma.

Marius was taken to the operating room once again,
and his pelvis was opened. To their dismay, his doctors

saw that the replacement kidney was badly swollen, and evidence of hemorrhage was present; the transplant would not survive. After the operation, the medical team attempted to save Marius by massive transfusion. Perhaps his blood might be cleansed by replacement, if it could not be filtered by a new kidney. Volunteers came from around Paris and donated blood. The transfusions helped Marius to recover somewhat, but it was not long before the toxic waste products began to accumulate again. He drifted into irreversible coma. On January 27, 1953, Marius Renard died. The immunologic barrier had not been bridged, even between mother and son.[1]

Human beings have an extraordinarily complex and adaptive array of defenses that shield us from injury, infection, cancer, and illness in general. This includes our immune barrier, whose cornerstone is the ability to recognize what is "foreign" from what is "ours," along with the power to target, isolate, and destroy the potentially harmful invader. Sadly, for Marius Renard, it was his mother's kidney—recognized as foreign—that became the target for destruction by his immune system. The very system that had evolved to protect the body from disease was now the adversary of advancing medical science. What the surgeons could well accomplish technically, the replacement of a diseased organ by a new one, was still being foiled by the body's extraordinary immune barrier.

Certainly our immune system did not evolve to prevent the transplanting of organs. Protection against this kind of invasion does not offer any advantage for survival of the species. Organ rejection after transplantation, rather, is a side-effect of the otherwise essential activity of protecting the body from viruses and cancers. As modern organ transplanters, it is our task to circumvent the body's immune barrier to the new or-

1. From *The Patients*, by Jurgen Thorwald (New York: Harcourt Brace Jovanovich, 1971). Quotation from p. 129.

gan, while keeping as intact as possible the body's vital defenses against disease. As we shall see in this and the following chapters, overcoming the immune barrier is not an easy job.

The immune system is but one part of the body's highly complex and varied defensive network. Our skin, for instance, shields out harmful ultraviolet light, holds in vital moisture, and simultaneously acts as a highly impenetrable barrier to microorganisms. The tiny hairs lining the breathing passages of the nose and lungs filter out airborne particles, such as dust, chemicals, and bacteria. Other barriers also exist to inhibit the onslaught of outside invaders.

Our ultimate defense is, however, the immune network, with its billions of microscopic cells and the even greater number of specialized chemical molecules they manufacture. Produced in the bone marrow and circulating throughout the bloodstream, the leukocytes, or white blood cells, are our final defense against disease. Although our understanding of their importance is modern, their name is derived from the ancient Greek: *leukos* for white and *kytos* for hollow container. The leukocytes can be subdivided by appearance and function into the "polys" (polymorphonuclear cells), "lymphs" (lymphocytes), "monos" (mononuclear cells), and "eos" (eosinophils). The job of each type of cell is highly specialized, yet working in concert they form one integrated system. Throughout the book we will discuss the roles of these vital cells in the transplant process, but for now, we will emphasize the special function of the lymphocytes and their impact on organ transplantation.

Lymphocytes

The lymphocytes normally make up only about 20 percent of the white blood cells circulating in the bloodstream. When stained with dye and viewed under the microscope, these cells have a large, centrally located blue nucleus, surrounded by a much smaller border of whitish cytoplasm.

Three special features are characteristic of these cells with regard to their effectiveness in the immune system (Table 2.1). First, they have *specificity*, which means that individual lymphocytes become activated only when they encounter their own particular target substance. For example, only a few lymphocytes become activated when we encounter the virus that causes measles; the rest of our lymphocytes remain quiet. Indeed, the purpose of the measles vaccine is to prime a few lymphocytes to recognize the specific measles virus. Should that virus present itself, these relatively few lymphocytes will be available to target the invader for destruction before it can cause infection. Fortunately, we have in our system many thousands of lymphocytes with specificity for most of the different foreign substances we may encounter day to day.

The second characteristic feature of the cells responsible for immunity is that they have *memory*. During World War II, as in earlier wars, extensive burns were common. Without intact skin to protect the body from fluid loss and invasion by infectious agents, death from a severe burn was inevitable. One attempted treatment was to use skin grafted from a healthy person to cover the burn victim.

But attempts to graft skin from one person to another failed. Indeed, while the initial replacement skin might take hold for about two weeks, a second graft of skin from the same donor evoked a much faster and more devastating rejection. Scientists now had clear evidence not only that the immune system recognizes the foreign invader, but that once so exposed remembers its prior encounter and reacts accordingly.

The body's rapid rejection of a second skin graft was termed

Table 2.1.   Special features of the immune system.

Specificity:	Each lymphocyte reacts only with its own target substance (virus, bacteria, tissue cell).
Memory:	The immune system responds more strongly the second time it encounters a target substance.
Tolerance:	The immune system distinguishes foreign target substances from our own cells and tissues.

the "second set response" by the British researchers Thomas Gibson and Sir Peter Medawar. It was already known that once the body encounters a foreign substance the lymphocytes will remember that exposure and be ready to react against it more vigorously a second time. This is what we mean when we say a person is immune to a virus, such as measles. The person's lymphocytes, which have previously encountered the virus, are ready to mount a rapid response should the same virus threaten again. Vaccination works by exposing a person to a weakened form of a virus, as a safe way to store in immunologic memory the capability to feud off possible future invasion. For organ transplantation, however, memory means that once exposed to foreign tissue, the body's lymphocytes will follow with a stronger rejection reaction the second time. Later in this chapter, when we discuss sensitization, we shall see how immunologic memory plays a critical role in organ rejection.

The third special feature of lymphocytes, termed *tolerance*, is the capacity of the immune system to distinguish between substances that make up our own bodies and those which come from outside. To keep our bodies from reacting against parts of themselves, the immune system eliminates all lymphocytes with specificity for ourselves, before they mature into functional cells that could produce damage. In human transplantation, the immune response to the replacement organ occurs because our lymphocytes recognize—as they should—that the new organ is not really part of ourselves. In other words, they are not tolerant to it. For a transplant to succeed without immunosuppressive drugs, it would be necessary for science to find a way to induce immunologic tolerance.

In the early 1950s a laboratory experiment demonstrated that this might someday be possible. Sir Peter Medawar had continued his interest in the immunology of skin grafts; ultimately he would receive the Nobel Prize for his efforts, particularly for demonstrating that the immunologic barrier to transplantation could be broken. As Medawar's experiments proceeded, he became increasingly interested in the potential role of age in the rejection process. He postulated that if, once sensitized, the adult's defenses provide immunity for life, perhaps there is a time early in life when the immune system can be bypassed so that it will accept foreign tissue in the future.

And so Medawar, along with his colleagues at University College, London, devised what has become a famous experiment in the history of science. They were expanding on an observation already made by an Australian researcher, Sir F. Macfarlane Burnet, who had shown that chicks developed tolerance to a virus if they were exposed to the virus before hatching. Medawar and his group took the concept a step further. They injected cells from Type B (brown) mice into newborn Type A (white) mice. When grown to maturity, these Type A mice would then accept a skin graft from a Type B mouse. Billingham, Brent, and Medawar termed this phenomenon "actively acquired tolerance." The discovery that the immunologic barrier could be breached was critical to the future of organ transplantation.

It should be pointed out that our lymphocytes are not always perfect in recognizing what is foreign from what is ours, and may mistakenly target our normal tissues for rejection. This is what occurs in the auto-immune diseases, such as rheumatoid arthritis and diabetes mellitus, among many others.

B and T Lymphocytes

Based on their essential functions, the immune system's lymphocytes can be divided into two major types, termed B and T cells. Although basically they have very different roles, they also can work in concert, an interplay that produces an enhanced result.

B cells manufacture *antibodies*, small Y-shaped molecules that float in the liquid portion of the bloodstream waiting to encounter foreign substances. One end of an antibody's chemical structure is devoted to a combining site capable of interacting only with a specific target substance, usually a potentially harmful foreign invader. It is the singular chemical makeup of a particular combining site that gives an antibody its remarkable degree of specificity. All the antibodies secreted by each individual B cell are identical and will interact only with the same target substance.

One of the ways in which we are protected from a variety of different biological threats is that our immune systems are capable of producing many thousands of different B cells. So, when we are exposed to the measles virus, we use B cells that make antibodies that react with the measles virus; when we are exposed to the polio virus, we use different B cells capable of secreting specific antibodies to counteract that virus, and so on. And, because the system has a memory, when we are exposed to a virus for which we have a specific B cell, that cell will swiftly produce many offspring B cells, which, in turn, will produce antibodies. For many viruses, a simple blood test can detect the presence of protective antibody, indicating prior exposure or inoculation and future potential immunity. So specific are these tests that we also can often monitor relatively recent exposure to a virus by noting a rising concentration of antibody in the bloodstream. The production of antibodies by B cells is called *humoral immunity*, from the Latin word *humor*, or liquid, because these biochemicals circulate in the fluid portion of the bloodstream.

The other basic type of lymphocytes, the T cells, are responsible for what is called *cellular immunity*. The name comes from the fact that the protective function of this type of immunity is based on the actions of the cell itself—either by direct contact of the T cell with its target, or by the T cell's ability to secrete molecules called *cytokines*, which neutralize the target cells around them. Using chemicals on their surfaces called *receptors*, T cells also have specificity. When a T cell receptor recognizes its target, the cell quickly begins to divide and multiply, thereby producing legions of offspring T cells, all of which have the same surface receptor and the same neutralizing capability against a specific target. Thus, after a first encounter with a foreign substance (antigen), for an entire lifetime our cellular defenses retain the capacity to mobilize quickly and efficiently against that particular invader. This is the memory function described earlier. Not surprisingly, both humoral and cellular immunity, which evolve to protect us from viral and bacterial infections, are critical in the body's efforts to reject a transplanted organ.

The immune system has many other components besides B and T cells that contribute to our defense against disease and that also contribute to the destruction of transplanted organs. For example, there are macrophages, cells that engulf foreign organisms, and there is the complement system, a group of molecules that can literally poke holes in the walls of cells to cause their destruction. But while these other components of the immune system help the B and T cells to cause graft destruction, none of them has the capacity to distinguish self from nonself tissues. Thus they depend on the B and T cells to tell them when to attack a transplanted organ.

On December 23, 1954, surgeons working at the Peter Bent Brigham Hospital (now the Brigham and Women's) in Boston performed the first successful kidney transplant. Instead of defeating the immune barrier, they did an end run around it, by transplanting a kidney from Ronald Herrick into his twin brother, Richard. Being identical twins, Ronald and Richard shared the same genetic structure, and hence the same proteins that define what is "self" from what is "foreign." Rejection did not occur. Richard lived with his transplanted kidney for eight years, and married the nurse who cared for him.

And then on May 24, 1956, the same surgical team repeated their success on Edith Helm, whose identical twin, Wanda, provided a kidney to save her sister. In only a few days after the operation, Edith looked and felt like a new person. The replacement kidney began virtually immediately to filter waste products. Edith's blood pressure dropped, her energy and appetite returned, and her vision, which had been blurring, returned to normal. A year and a half later, to her doctors' dismay, Edith

Helm was pregnant. But to their surprise the pregnancy had no ill effects on Edith's transplanted kidney. In March of 1958, Edith Helm became the first transplant recipient to give birth. "I had a name for a girl," she said, "but hadn't really picked one for a boy, so we ended up naming him after the doctor, John Merrill."[2]

Antigens

The substances that trigger B and T cells to work are protein substances called *antigens*. In order to accomplish this triggering, an antigen must be the right size and chemical shape to fit—much like a key in a lock—into either the recognition site of an antibody or the receptor site of a T cell. Whole cells, such as bacteria, are too large to be recognized by the immune system. Instead, the activators are proteins called *surface antigens*, which reside on the outside of the cell. Even viruses, which are much smaller than bacteria, are too large to be recognized. Indeed, only small fragments of the total structure of a virus serve as stimulating antigens to trigger the working of the B and T cells.

Transplantation Antigens

When transplanted organs are rejected, it is because the recipient's immune system recognizes that the surface antigens on the replacement organ do not match his or her own surface antigens. Lacking tolerance for these proteins, the recipient's B and T cells become stimulated, generating the rejection process.

It is significant that, to some extent, our B and T cells are capable of recognizing different antigens. B cells, for example, can pick out the antigens that define our blood groups—so if a person with type O blood were given a kidney from a person with type A blood, there would be a humoral, but not a cellular, immune response.

2. From *The Patients*, by Jurgen Thorwald (New York: Harcourt Brace Jovanovich, 1971). Quotation from p. 143.

On the other hand, both B and T cells recognize a set of proteins called *transplantation antigens* or *histocompatibility antigens*. Histocompatibility, another medical word derived from the ancient Greek, comes from *histos,* for web or tissue, and means "tissue compatibility." There are two broad categories of histocompatibility antigens, *major* and *minor.* As their names imply, the major antigens are especially important in causing organ rejection. When we say, "We have a match," we mean we have found a donor and a recipient whose tissues bear many identical major histocompatibility antigens.

The major histocompatibility antigens are determined (the scientific word is "encoded") by our basic genetic structure. Located on a very small segment of the DNA within our chromosomes in the nucleus of our cells, they confer an individual's major histocompatibility complex, abbreviated MHC. Every animal species has its own unique MHC antigens; in humans they are called HLA antigens. Though histocompatibility antigens were identified first by their ability to evoke cellular immunity, they generally also stimulate B cells to produce specific antibodies. B cells produce no humoral response, however, to minor histocompatibility antigens.

There are a number of different HLA antigens on the surface of each human cell. These can be grouped into two principal types, called class I and class II antigens, each with its own subcategories. The class I type has A, B, and C antigens and the class II type has DR, DQ, and DP antigens. Thus, there are six types of HLA antigens encoded by the genes of the major histocompatibility complex. But, because we inherit half our genes from each biological parent, every human being has twelve different HLA antigens on the surface of his or her cells. And, to complicate the situation further, the number of variations of the genes in the human species that determine (that is, encode) any particular HLA antigen is very large. For example, there are at least thirty different forms of the gene that encodes just the HLA A antigen. Now that many of the antigens have been identified and given numbers, it is possible to "HLA type" a person to see which HLA antigens he or she expresses. For example, someone might be found to express HLA A3 and A27 (one antigen inherited from each parent), HLA B6 and B22, HLA DR2 and DR4, and so on. It is rather like genetic bingo. In practice, it is not yet possible to identify all twelve of the HLA antigens, so currently we usually talk about the HLA type of six antigens, two each of the A, B, and DR types.

Because there are so many possible HLA A antigens that an individual may have, and since there are other additional HLA antigens as well, the number of possible combinations of HLA antigens any one person might express is enormous. It is thus very unusual to find two *unrelated* persons with exactly the same HLA type. The expression that someone is "one in a million" is nearly true for transplantation.

But, because we inherit half of our genes from each parent, the chances of achieving partial or complete HLA matching within a family are much better. Each parent and child pair is a one-haplotype, or haplo-identical, match (*haplo* means half). However, two siblings may be fully identical for major HLA antigens, if both inherit the same HLA structure. Identical twins, like Richard and Ronald Herrick and Edith and Wanda Helm, have a further advantage of matching both the major and minor HLA antigens, because they have the exact same genetic structure.

On the other hand, siblings may inherit only one shared gene, leaving them with the same one-haplotype situation as parent and child. Or, for a pair of siblings, both haplotypes may be different, so that the siblings are HLA-unmatched. This will be discussed again in Chapter 9 on bone marrow transplantation, where HLA matching is especially critical.

While the major histocompatibility antigens are very important and quite complicated, the minor histocompatibility antigens are easier, perhaps because we know very little about them. There are approximately fifty of these antigens, and most of them have yet to be named. Only in identical twins are they matched. Fortunately, the minor histocompatibility antigens cause relatively weak rejection reactions that can generally be suppressed with currently available drugs.

The Immune Response to Transplanted Organs

To date, three principal kinds of immune responses to transplanted organs have been identified, and there are probably others that are not yet so well understood. Two of these responses involve humoral immunity, while the third involves cellular immunity (see Table 2.2).

Hyperacute Rejection

Hyperacute rejection is a humoral response that occurs when a recipient already has a large number of antibodies circulating in the bloodstream that react with antigens on the donor organ. These may be antibodies that react with the blood group antigens (ABO antibodies), or they may react with the HLA antigens of the donor organ. ABO antibodies come into play if the donor and the recipient have incompatible blood types, while antibodies to HLA antigens may exist if a recipient has had a previous encounter with HLA antigens from another person—by transfusion, pregnancy, or a prior transplant. These antibodies arise from a process called *sensitization*, and we say the person is sensitized. If a transplant is performed in a sensitized recipient—that is, one whose blood already has antibodies that react with the donor—the transplanted organ will suffer virtually instantaneous hyperacute rejection. In these cases, the transplanted organ will not even survive to

Table 2.2. Immune response to transplanted organs.

Type of rejection	Mechanism	Time course
Hyperacute	B cells	Almost instantaneous
Acute	T cells	Usually during the early weeks
Chronic	B cells	Generally over years

the end of the surgery. There is currently no treatment for hyperacute rejection, so strict precautions must be taken to avoid performing transplants when the recipient has antibodies to the donor organ. Nowadays hyperacute rejection rarely occurs, because every recipient is tested for sensitization to the prospective donor's antigens before surgery.

Acute Rejection

In the absence of preexisting hostile antibodies, most transplanted organs survive without any evidence of immunologic attack during the first several days after surgery. This is because it takes time for unsensitized lymphocytes to recognize that the replacement organ is foreign, and to mount an immune response against it. However, between five and ten days after transplantation, the recipient's T cells begin to respond to the donor organ's histocompatibility antigens. The injury caused by this cellular immune response is called *acute rejection.* Without medical treatment in the form of immunosuppression (see Chapter 3) to block the T cell response, every transplanted organ (except those between identical twins) would be rejected within about two weeks. Even with our most sophisticated tools to suppress the normal immune response, about one week after surgery most transplanted organs undergo some acute rejection, which causes diminished function. Additional immunosuppressive treatment must then be given to halt the rejection process, or the replacement organ will be lost. Fortunately, most of these episodes can be reversed, so that the transplanted organ returns to normal function. Nevertheless, despite vigorous treatment, a few patients suffer such severe acute rejection that their organ is permanently rejected. Somewhat more commonly, some recipients undergo several episodes of acute rejection in the early period after transplantation. While these episodes are both frightening and frustrating to patients and their families, for the majority of new recipients treatment is successful and their transplant can be saved.

Even with successful immunosuppressive treatment during

the first several weeks after surgery, the body's T cells continue to be stimulated by the replacement organ's foreign histocompatibility antigens. On the positive side, the likelihood that they will become activated and begin to reject the transplanted organ diminishes gradually over time. This means that as the months go by after surgery, the amount of immunosuppression needed to prevent rejection can be reduced. Nonetheless, acute rejection episodes are always a possibility, even years after transplantation. Recipients must, therefore, continue to take immunosuppressive medication for as long as they have their replacement organ.

Chronic Rejection

The third type of immune response to transplanted organs occurs over a relatively long period of time after the transplant, and thus is called *chronic rejection*. Often seemingly caused by humoral immunity—perhaps because our medical tools for blocking B cells are more limited than for T cells—chronic rejection manifests itself as slow deterioration of the transplanted organ despite increasing doses of immunosuppression. Fortunately, most recipients do not encounter this problem.

Matching Donor and Recipient

Since the immune response to transplanted organs is triggered by the donor organ's antigens, one might predict that finding a donor and a recipient whose antigens are closely matched would decrease the magnitude of the rejection process. In some cases this turns out to be true, while in others the beneficial effect is less obvious.

ABO Blood Group Compatibility

Antigen matching is very important in the case of blood groups. Every human being has one of four basic blood group types: O, A, B, or AB. Blood group is determined by the A and B antigens residing on the surface of the red blood cells (and certain other tissues). People with group A blood express the A antigen, those with group B express the B antigen, those with group AB express both A and B, and those with group O blood do not express either. It is a peculiar feature of the blood group system that people have antibodies in their blood against the blood group antigens that they do not express, even if they have never been exposed to antigens from other blood groups. Thus O individuals have antibodies to A and B antigens, A individuals have antibodies to B antigens, B individuals have antibodies to A antigens, and AB individuals do not have antibodies. Antibodies against blood group antigens are capable of causing hyperacute rejection of many organs. As summarized in Table 2.3, people in blood group O cannot receive organs from either A or B donors; A recipients cannot receive transplants from B or AB donors; B recipients cannot receive transplants from A or AB donors; and AB recipients are able to receive organs from donors in any blood group. Donors who are acceptable for a given recipient from the point of view of their blood group antigens are called ABO-compatible. ABO compatibility is important in the transplantation of all organs except the liver, since this organ seems to be unusually resistant to hyperacute rejection and humoral immunity. And even in liver transplantation, blood group compatibility is probably helpful.

HLA Matching of Related Living Donors

When performing a kidney transplant it is possible to obtain the donor organ from a living person, since human beings

Table 2.3. The ABO blood group system.

Blood group	% of population	Antigens expressed	Antibodies expressed	Potential organ donors
O	47%	None	anti-A, anti-B	O
A	42%	A	anti-B	O,A
B	8%	B	anti-A	O,B
AB	3%	AB	None	O,A,B,AB

have two kidneys but only need one to maintain normal function. Recall that the first successful kidney transplant was performed using the kidney of an identical twin. If the living donor is a family member, it is possible that some, or all, of the HLA antigens will match. As we explained earlier, parents and their children always share half, but generally not more, of their HLA antigens. Siblings may share none, half, or all of their HLA antigens, depending on whether they inherit the same or different histocompatibility genes from their two parents. In transplanting a kidney from one family member to another, there are significant advantages to better matching of HLA antigens. HLA identical kidney transplants have about a 95 percent chance of organ survival one year after surgery, HLA half-matched (haplo-identical) kidneys have about a 90 percent chance of surviving after one year, and unmatched kidneys have about an 85 percent chance. Therefore, if there are several possible family members who could be an organ donor, it is preferable to use the better match. In fact, kidneys from family members who are completely HLA unmatched generally do not survive any better than organs from unrelated, cadaveric (deceased) donors. In such situations, it is usually not suggested that family members act as donors.

Knowing that good HLA matches often require less immunosuppression and have fewer complications overall, before considering a potential donor and recipient transplant teams run tests to determine all of the major histocompatibility antigens. Even with the best match available, donor and recipient will still be unmatched for many minor histocompatibility antigens, so some immunosuppression will be required. Only organ transplants between identical twins, all of whose antigens are identical, can survive without any immunosuppression.

HLA Matching of Cadaveric Donors

Many (probably about one-half to two-thirds) of the organs used for transplantation come from donors who have recently become brain-dead (and hence are called *cadaveric*), but whose other organs continue to function well. It is possible to type and compare the HLA antigens of these donors and compare them with those of the many possible recipients waiting for transplants. Available organs can thus be distributed on the basis of the HLA match.

The benefit of using this system to distribute cadaveric donors has been studied extensively and remains controversial. It appears that HLA matching between donor and recipient produces some statistical advantage with regard to the success of the transplant, but most of this advantage is seen only if *all* identified HLA antigens are identical. Unfortunately, it is not easy to find such a match.

There is a national computer system that lists the HLA antigens of every person in North America awaiting kidney transplantation, and similar registries exist in Europe and Japan. When a donor organ becomes available, its HLA type is compared to the list. When a perfect match is possible, a special effort is made to provide that kidney to that recipient. It helps that kidneys can be transported across the country (while the heart, for instance, can be maintained outside of the donor for only a few hours), since because of the complexity of the HLA system a matching donor and recipient are rarely found in close geographic proximity. Thus, among the solid organs, HLA matching currently is practical only for kidneys. As we discuss later, HLA matching is very important in bone marrow transplantation, and is feasible because bone marrow is taken from a living donor, who can travel to a hospital near the recipient.

Crossmatch Testing

Because hyperacute rejection is untreatable, it is important to avoid transplanting an organ when it might occur. Therefore, transplant teams avoid putting an organ into a recipient who has antibodies that will react with the donor's cells. As already mentioned, one way to ensure this does not happen is to determine compatibility by blood group. A second method is to test for the presence of antibodies that react in the HLA system, a test called a *crossmatch*. This test is performed in the tissue-typing laboratory by mixing a small blood sample from the prospective recipient with lymphocyte cells from the potential donor. If, after combining, the donor's cells die, the crossmatch is termed positive. This means the recipient has antibodies that are reacting to the antigens on the surface of the donor's cells. Although we say "positive," this means that a transplant cannot be performed, because it would result in hyperacute rejection and organ failure.

Whenever a donor organ becomes available, a crossmatch is set up to screen blood samples from many possible recipients. Only those with negative crossmatches are considered further as recipients for that organ. Since, depending on many factors, the level of antibodies in a person's bloodstream changes over time (see the next section on sensitization), it is important to test a recently obtained blood sample. Therefore, someone awaiting kidney transplantation will send blood regularly—usually about once a month—to a tissue-typing laboratory where crossmatches can be performed. These blood specimens will be frozen and saved, so that a repeat test can be made each time a new potential donor becomes available.

Sensitization

When a crossmatch is positive, the recipient is said to be *sensitized* to that donor. In fact, this only means that the recipient's B cells are sensitized, because the crossmatch solely measures humoral immunity. As yet, we do not have an easy way to measure T cell sensitization. Fortunately, T cell sensitization does not appear to have the same critical implications for successful transplantation as B cell sensitization.

For patients awaiting an organ transplant, there are two important principles regarding sensitization. The first is to prevent it whenever possible. Unfortunately, preventing sensitization is difficult because we cannot control most of the factors that produce it. Exposure to foreign HLA antigens occurs when women bear children, when people receive blood transfusions, and of course, with organ transplantation. While some persons may experience exposure without becoming sensitized, it is generally the case that the most highly sensitized recipients have had several different types of contact with HLA antigens. Among these factors, only the administration of blood transfusions can be directly controlled while people await transplantation. Therefore, doctors consider the risks of sensitization before administering blood to a potential candidate for organ replacement.

The second principle is to keep careful track of the level of sensitization of prospective recipients. Blood from all potential recipients in a geographic area is periodically tested against a panel of cells obtained from many different volunteers selected because together they express most of the known human HLA antigens. Dozens of separate crossmatches are done for each recipient, and hundreds of recipients are tested each month. If the blood of an individual recipient does not kill any of the cells in the panel, that recipient is said to be *unsensitized*. Someone whose blood kills 50 percent of the cells in the panel is 50 percent sensitized. Some potential recipients have antibodies that kill all of the cells in the panel; they are 100 percent sensitized. Obviously, it is easier to find a donor organ for someone who is unsensitized than for someone who is highly sensitized. Since the HLA types represented in the test panel are known, it is often possible to identify the particular HLA antigens to which a prospective recipient already has antibodies. Once this is accomplished, it is possible to eliminate many prospective recipients from further consideration, even before a crossmatch is done. The remaining candidates can then be tested by crossmatching, to make certain they are not sensitized to that particular donor.

The level of sensitization is sometimes a factor in distributing kidneys. Since it is hard to find a donor who is crossmatch-negative for a highly sensitized candidate, such candidates have a high priority when a compatible organ becomes available. In practice, the more highly sensitized candidates wait longer than unsensitized persons to receive a kidney transplant. Occasionally, however, serendipity works in their favor—just the right organ becomes available shortly after they go on the list, and they are given priority status for it. But, unfortunately, some very highly sensitized candidates wait years for a compatible organ.

Blood Transfusions

Since transfusions are one way people become sensitized to foreign HLA antigens, doctors used to go to great lengths to avoid giving blood products to potential transplant patients. But when the issue was carefully studied, it was learned that transplants had a better success rate in patients who had received blood transfusions, and who later were transplanted with a negative crossmatch, than in recipients who had never been transfused. In other words, while transfusions increase the risk of sensitization—potentially delaying the time when a recipient will receive a transplant—they also improve the survival of the transplanted organ when it finally becomes available. This phenomenon, although seemingly an accurate medical fact, appears to contradict what we have otherwise said about transplant immunology.

The reasons for this outcome are complicated, and are still not entirely understood. Nevertheless, in the face of medical data suggesting a beneficial effect of exposing candidates to antigens via the transfusion process, many transplant groups around the country began giving blood transfusions to prospective organ recipients—even if they did not otherwise need them. More recently, the perspective is changing again, especially in light of our improved ability to manipulate the immune system to accept a transplanted organ. Moreover, partly because of the AIDS epidemic, the potential risks of blood transfusion are being emphasized. Even though the risk of transmitting AIDS by blood transfusions is now almost entirely avoidable, other less dangerous but still harmful viruses, such as the one that causes hepatitis, can be contracted this way. In addition, with the recent availability of erythropoietin, in the form of a drug called EPO, which stimulates the bone marrow to make more blood cells even while people are on dialysis, the need for transfusions has been reduced. Overall, the balance between the risks and benefits of administering blood now seems to be much closer. Many transplant groups rarely provide intentional transfusions to transplant candidates. Currently, the transplant recipient and his or her physician should handle this question on an individual basis.

Most of our knowledge of the immune system's response to transplanted organs has been achieved within the past thirty years. As we reflect upon our own field, the pace at which new information is being garnered seems staggering. The early forms of immunosuppression for preventing organ rejection were found by trial and error. But increasingly, through advances in the science of immunology, we are proceeding down a more deliberate path to better ways for blocking the immune barrier. Thus, basic research leads the way to applications that ultimately improve the lives of people who need organ replacement.

3

Immunosuppression

The headline in the *Chicago Sun-Times* on June 19, 1950,
said "Woman Dies, Kidney May Save Life of 2nd."

"A healthy kidney was removed from the body of a
dead woman and used to replace the diseased kidney of
a dying woman in a historic 90-minute operation by two
teams of doctors in Little Company of Mary Hospital."

But the *Chicago Tribune* reported on May 23, 1951:
"The first attempt in history to transplant a kidney from
one human to another has ended in failure . . . Inability
of tissues of one person to be compatible when transplanted to another was given as the reason for the failure. The committee, composed of top experts in the field,
pledged that no more such operations be attempted until
science uncovers new knowledge about the biological
compatibility of tissues and organs."

These are newspaper accounts of Ruth Tucker, who
on June 17, 1950, became the first person to receive a
transplanted kidney. The donor was another woman of
identical blood type and almost identical age. Within
minutes of the operation, the surgeons were hopeful,
as even on the operating table the replacement organ
showed signs of life. The days progressed and hope increased. The new kidney made urine and Ruth's energy

improved. Not long after, she was discharged from the hospital to her home. By November of that year, *JAMA*—the *Journal of the American Medical Association*—was reporting the apparent success of the incredible operation. By mid-winter, however, Ruth Tucker began to notice that her urinary output was diminishing. Her doctors hoped the cause was no more than a mechanical obstruction that could be relieved. They performed another operation. After exposing the replacement kidney to view, they quickly realized why so little urine was being produced: the transplanted kidney had shrunk dramatically; Mrs. Tucker's body had rejected the foreign organ. The first human transplant in the modern medical era had not been a success.[1]

Ruth Tucker's pioneering story illustrates what, until recently, was an inviolable rule of human biology: every organ transplanted from a donor other than an identical twin will elicit an immune response in the recipient. Unless blocked with immunosuppression, this normal biological process will, in short order, produce rejection of the replacement organ. It is, therefore, also a rule that for as long as a recipient has a replacement organ, he or she will have to take medications to suppress the immune response. The success of modern organ transplantation is in large part the result of our newly developed ability to block the rejection of the new organ while still maintaining adequate immune function to protect the body from infection and disease.

A Delicate Balance

Immunosuppression can be divided into two kinds. *Specific suppression* blocks the immune response to only one or a few

1. From *The Patients*, by Jurgen Thorwald (New York: Harcourt Brace Jovanovich, 1971). Quotations from pp. 97–100.

antigens, leaving the response to other antigens intact. *Non-specific suppression* blocks the immune response to all foreign antigens more or less equally. Obviously, it would be preferable for transplant recipients to receive specific immunosuppression that would block only their response to the antigens of their donor organ. But while specific immunosuppression can be accomplished in a variety of ways in experimental animals, none has yet been found to work well in humans. Clearly, achieving this goal holds great promise for the future of organ transplantation.

Nonspecific immunosuppression requires a delicate balance between the conflicting needs to prevent organ rejection and to maintain adequate defenses against infection. Fortunately, the amount of immunosuppression needed to preserve a healthy transplanted organ decreases after the first several months following surgery. Therefore, most recipients can keep their transplants with a dose of immunosuppression that allows them to carry out normal lives—working, for example, even in highly contagious environments like hospitals or schools—without hiding from the world in a plastic bubble. But even years after transplant surgery some immunosuppression is still necessary.

If recipients skip some of their doses, or if their medication is reduced to too low a level, they may experience rejection even years after receiving their transplant. More immunosuppression is then necessary in the short run to avoid total organ failure, and this increased dosage may even be needed over the long term. Thus, the effort to achieve a low dose of immunosuppression sometimes may backfire, leading instead to higher doses and the problems that can result from these drugs.

In addition to lowering the body's defenses against disease, all the current immunosuppressive drugs have the potential to cause side-effects and complications. Moreover, each specific medicine has its own range of possible side-effects, and individuals vary in their reaction to these drugs. Experience has shown that it is possible to minimize the toxicity of immunosuppressives by taking a number of different drugs at the same time. Using a combination of drugs reduces the adverse effects of each medicine, while accomplishing a sufficient overall level of immunosuppression.

There is, as yet, no mix that is best for every patient. While we will describe each drug in more detail later in this chapter, the important point is that the specific regimen of immuno-suppressives must be tailored for the individual. One recipient, for example, may have high blood pressure on cyclosporine, and thus require less cyclosporine compensated by more pred-nisone. Another may not tolerate azathioprine, but may have no difficulty with a relatively high dose of cyclosporine. During the months after transplantation, most recipients make fre-quent follow-up visits to the transplant team to adjust and readjust their mix of medicines.

Steroids

It was in 1936 that scientists working independently in the United States and Switzerland discovered cortisone, one of the vital steroids produced by the body's adrenal glands. Hailed as a miracle drug, by the 1950s cortisone was being used in almost any disease when no other treatment was available. It soon became clear that steroids possess an incredible power to alter—indeed to suppress—normal immune function. And so, it was not long before they were employed by the organ trans-planters.

There are several different types of steroids, including pred-nisone, an oral form of the medicine, and methylprednisolone (Solu-Medrol), which is usually administered intravenously. Other types of steroids exist as well, including a variety of anabolic steroids sometimes misused by athletes. These are quite different, however, and are not used for immunosuppres-sion.

Although steroids are essential for a healthy life and hence are manufactured by the body under ordinary circumstances, when used for immunosuppression they must be given in much larger amounts than normally produced by our adrenal glands. Taking steroid medication over a long period of time gradually reduces a person's capacity to produce these substances. Eventually it may be lost altogether. A person who suddenly stops taking steroids may become very sick, suffering from what is called adrenal insufficiency, a type of steroid withdrawal that can be fatal.

Patients who take steroids must realize that it may be necessary to adjust their dosage from time to time. For instance, the usual dose recipients take for immunosuppression may not be sufficient to cope with periods of unusual physiological stress, such as surgery or serious illness. In these situations we usually administer extra doses of steroids in the form of hydrocortisone (Solu-Cortef), an intravenous, short-acting form of the drug. Another feature of steroids relates to the fact that their manufacture is influenced naturally by the body's circadian, or twenty-four-hour, rhythm. Thus, the time during the day in which these substances are taken makes a difference. Normally, steroids are produced in highest concentration early in the morning, followed by a gradual decline throughout the day. Therefore, steroid medicines should also be taken primarily in the morning. When they are taken in large doses in the evening, it is common to feel restless and uncomfortable through the night, and other unpleasant side-effects may also arise.

Although after half a century of intensive research we still do not fully understand how steroids accomplish immunosuppression, we have, over the years, learned to use them to achieve our ends. In practice, steroids are generally administered to transplant patients in three different ways. First, right after surgery, they are given in fairly high doses intravenously (a typical dose is 200 milligrams per day), and then orally, to ensure acceptance of the graft. This is called the *induction period*, and steroids are particularly helpful in this period because they start working almost immediately. In the past, these high doses had to be maintained for months after the transplant. More recently, the availability of cyclosporine and other new drugs has made it possible to rather quickly diminish the oral dose of prednisone. Second, oral prednisone is used at a much reduced dose—usually only between 15 and 20 milligrams per day—as *maintenance therapy*. Third, high "pulse" doses in the range of 500 milligrams of methylprednisolone (Solu-Medrol) are given intravenously to abort rejection episodes. Occasionally the pulse treatment can also be accomplished by a short period of relatively high doses of oral prednisone. If several steroid pulses fail to reverse rejection, other forms of therapy are required.

Side-Effects

As the proponents of the steroid "miracle" learned in the 1950s, these drugs have many potential side-effects. Aside from the decreased immunity that occurs with all forms of nonspecific immunosuppression, short-term side-effects of high doses of steroids include:

- Mood changes, ranging from a "high" to agitation and confusion, and in some cases feelings of depression.

- Suppression of the normal fever response and other manifestations of infection.

- Elevation of blood sugar, particularly in patients who already have diabetes.

Over the longer term, the side-effects of steroids tend to be related to the total maintenance dose required, so that, depending on their dosage, some people may experience the following effects:

- A shift in the distribution of their body fat so that their cheeks become puffy and their back develops a rounded appearance. These are referred to as Cushingoid features, after Dr. Harvey Cushing, who first described the pattern in people with excess steroid production from hyperactive adrenal glands.

- Thinning and weakness of their bones, which may cause a hip problem called "aseptic necrosis" or a hip fracture. A few patients eventually require artificial hip replacement. For this reason, we suggest that transplant recipients use an exercise bicycle or swim for exercise, rather than jog, to avoid strain on their bones.

- An increased tendency toward high blood pressure. Dietary restriction of salt and fat can help avoid this problem.

- A decrease in skin thickness with a resulting susceptibility to easy bruising.

- Diabetes, which may require medication by mouth or insulin by injection.

- Increased development of cataracts over time.

- Some increase in acne or facial hair growth.

It should be emphasized that with the relatively low doses of prednisone now used to prevent rejection, these adverse side-effects are much less common than they were in the past.

One effect experienced by almost everyone taking prednisone is a dramatic increase in appetite. Weight gain is, therefore, a serious long-term problem for many transplant recipients. This is a psychological problem as well as a physical one, since virtually no one in our culture likes being overweight. It is also a source of medical concern, since obesity can cause or aggravate many conditions common in Western society: heart disease, hypertension, diabetes, arthritis, and so on. Transplant recipients should therefore work over time with hospital dietary staff to develop strategies for maintaining normal weight.

Another fairly common side-effect of prednisone is irritation of the stomach lining. If preventive measures are not taken, the inflammation can progress to gastric or duodenal ulcers with intestinal bleeding. Therefore, antacids are usually prescribed to be taken on a regular basis, especially when it is necessary to take relatively high doses of steroids.

The most insidious side-effect of prednisone is that its non-specific immunosuppressive action may block one's normal physiological responses to infection. Thus, a person taking prednisone may have a viral infection without experiencing fever or the other customary signs of the illness. For example, a viral infection of the liver, which in a normal person would be recognized, in an immunosuppressed person might take years to show its effect. Unfortunately, during that time there could be irreversible damage to the organ. For this reason, medical teams perform regular physical examinations, including blood tests, to detect possible low-level, chronic infection.

A full list of side-effects associated with steroids would go on much longer. These other side-effects, however, are less common than the ones already discussed. As mentioned previously, one of the recent dramatic and positive changes in the field of organ transplantation has been the ability to decrease the administration of prednisone. In turn, this has meant a significant reduction in the frequency of steroid-related side-effects. Nevertheless, anyone taking these drugs should promptly report to his or her doctor any unpleasant or unusual physical symptom, as these medications can produce a wide array of potential side-effects.

Azathioprine (Imuran)

A second drug frequently used for immunosuppression is aza-thioprine (marketed as Imuran), which interferes with the ability of cells to divide. Azathioprine is also a nonspecific immunosuppressive. It is effective in the transplant setting because when responding to foreign antigens cells of the immune system divide very frequently.

Not all transplant recipients receive azathioprine. Some start taking it months after surgery, when the dose of other medicines has been reduced. It also may be helpful as an alternative—when the side-effects of another medicine require finding a different combination of immunosuppressives.

After transplantation, a typical dose of azathioprine is 100 milligrams per day, taken either orally or intravenously. The intravenous dose is, of course, usually limited to the hospital setting. Adjustments in the dose may be needed for each individual. Since all bone marrow cells divide frequently, they are also susceptible to the effects of azathioprine. It is therefore necessary to take frequent blood cell counts, until a stable dose of the drug is achieved. If the blood counts are low, the patient may have to stop taking this medicine for a while to give the bone marrow time to recover.

Because it is nonspecific in its action, azathioprine has many potential side-effects, including:

- Thinning of the hair.
- Skin lesions, including skin cancers.
- Abnormalities of the uterine cervix (called cervical dysplasia, which can be detected by regular PAP smears and then treated).
- Abnormal liver function.
- Serious impairment of bone marrow function when azathioprine is taken in combination with allopurinol (Zyloprim), a medication used to treat gout.

While this list may be worrisome, it is important to note that the frequency of these adverse side-effects is relatively low. Azathioprine has been used to prevent rejection for more than thirty-five years, and for most people, it has been safe at the low doses required to inhibit organ rejection.

Cyclosporine (Sandimmune)

Originally called Cyclosporin A, cyclosporine or CsA, a relatively recent addition to the group of medicines we use to prevent rejection, has proven to be one of the most significant advances to date in the field of organ replacement. Indeed, its discovery has been largely responsible for an enormous increase in the number of transplants being performed and the success of these operations. Especially in the fields of heart and liver replacement, both long- and short-term survival have improved dramatically with the introduction of cyclosporine.

The immunosuppressive effect of cyclosporine seems to involve blocking T cells from sending and receiving some of the signals they require for activation. Its principal effect is thus on cellular immunity, although it may also have some impact on B cell immunity because there seems to be interaction between T and B cells that helps B cells to respond to foreign antigens.

Taking CsA

Cyclosporine can be given orally or intravenously, but the two routes are not equivalent, as only one-third of the dose is required when CsA is administered directly into the bloodstream. However, the greater efficiency of the intravenous preparation is a mixed blessing, as it is much more apt to produce kidney damage, seizures, and other neurologic problems. Therefore, we try, whenever possible, to avoid using intravenous CsA, preferring the oral form even if it must be administered via a tube introduced into the stomach during times when patients are unable to drink. The oral form of CsA also requires careful preparation, since it is chemically unstable when exposed to light for prolonged periods. It also will stick to plastic. And, because cyclosporine is an oily liquid, it does not dissolve well in water. To overcome these drawbacks, patients who take CsA are advised to follow these directions:

1. Measure accurately the prescribed amount by drawing it up in a syringe with measured markings along the side (each milliliter of liquid contains 100 milligrams of CsA).

2. Place the CsA in a glass or ceramic mug.

3. Mix thoroughly with chocolate milk or apple juice (cyclosporine can also be mixed with many other liquids), and drink.

Cyclosporine is now also available in capsule form, which is easier for some patients to take than the liquid preparation. However, the capsules are large, and some patients find them unpleasant.

Since cyclosporine is not absorbed in the stomach, but rather further down the gut, taking it with a meal speeds its absorption. The presence of food stimulates intestinal motion and hence absorption of the CsA into the bloodstream.

It takes many doses to build up in the body the level of cyclosporine that will prevent rejection. Therefore, patients begin by taking relatively high doses of CsA, which are tapered over time to a lower maintenance level. The beginning dose is approximately 12 milligrams for each kilogram of body weight, and this is typically halved over the long term to about 6 milligrams per kilogram. (One kilogram is approximately 2.2 pounds.) It usually takes many weeks to taper the CsA down to a maintenance level. Some transplant recipients are able to prevent rejection with an even lower dose. When relatively high doses are needed, the daily dose is usually divided in half: one half taken in the morning, one half in the evening. At lower doses it can all be taken once each morning. The speed with which the dose can be decreased to maintenance levels is rather variable among recipients, even those receiving the same type of transplant.

The concentration of cyclosporine circulating in the body can be measured with a blood test, and the results used to decide when and how to adjust the dose taken. But blood levels alone are not sufficient, since some patients experience side-effects (see next page) at relatively low concentrations, while others seem to have insufficient immunosuppression even when their levels are relatively high. Therefore, each person's dose of CsA will be adjusted individually according to laboratory results, manifestation of side-effects, and functioning of the transplant.

Cyclosporine is an expensive medicine, costing as much as six thousand dollars for a year's supply. Many recipients' medications are covered in full, or in large part, by their insurance or through special state funds, but for others the cost of cyclosporine is an important problem in their life after a successful transplant has been achieved.

Potential Side-Effects

While cyclosporine has been an invaluable addition to our battery of medications for preventing rejection, it is also a difficult drug for both recipients and physicians to use effectively. This is because CsA may produce a variety of serious potential side-effects, which can occur at almost the same dose that is required to achieve adequate immunosuppression. In other words, there often is a relatively narrow range of dosing in which the medication will both prevent rejection and be tolerated by the body.

The most common potentially serious side-effect of CsA is on the kidneys. In the short term, cyclosporine frequently causes reduced kidney function, which can be measured readily by blood tests for BUN (blood urea nitrogen) and creatinine. These two waste products, which are produced normally by the body, rise to abnormal levels when the kidney is functioning poorly in the face of CsA toxicity. Fortunately, the toxic side-effects usually abate when the dose of CsA is reduced. Over the longer term, CsA can cause scarring of the kidneys, producing chronic damage that may not be reversed even if the dose taken is lowered.

Sometimes, it is difficult to tell whether a kidney recipient's reduced organ function is due to too much CsA or to rejection of the kidney transplant. If the problem is drug side-effects, the dose must be lowered, while if the difficulty is rejection, the medication should be increased. Adjusting to these circumstances requires experience and careful assessment, often including a kidney biopsy. To date, the biopsy is our most accurate tool to distinguish between CsA toxicity and kidney rejection.

Other side-effects of cyclosporine may also arise. While no one patient is likely to experience all or even most of them, it is important to be aware of—and be able to recognize and communicate to your doctor—the side-effects listed below. CsA may, for instance, produce:

- Elevated blood pressure (hypertension), sufficient to require medical treatment.

- A rise in blood levels of potassium. While this is usually of little consequence, it should be monitored with periodic blood tests.

- Minor thickening of the gingiva (gums).

- Increased hair growth, usually in areas of the body where hair is not wanted (unfortunately, not in the area of male-pattern baldness). This can be a sensitive emotional issue for some, particularly teenagers and young women. Your physician, or a dermatologist, can suggest ways to deal with this cosmetic problem.

- Mild abnormalities of liver function, usually noted only on blood testing. Since these can sometimes be significant, we perform periodic blood tests to monitor liver function.

- Shakiness of the hands, called a tremor. Some patients describe a sensation of "the jitters," or a feeling of being confined or "cooped-up."

- Seizures, the most serious neurologic side-effect.

Most of these side-effects of CsA can be avoided, or reduced to an easily tolerated level, if the dose taken is decreased. The amount taken must be lowered slowly and carefully, however, to avoid setting off a rejection episode. The important message is that transplant recipients, like anyone taking medication, should be aware of the potential side-effects of the drugs they are taking. Be sure to report to your physician promptly any troubling sign or symptom.

Finally, cyclosporine, like all of the immunosuppressives currently available, increases *slightly* the risk of developing cancer, especially B cell lymphoma. Fortunately, the B cells usually return to normal if the CsA dose is decreased. Over time, however, a true cancer of the B cell system, which can be fatal, may develop. Again, while the chance of developing cancer is present for anyone on immunosuppression, this risk is actually very small (less than 3 percent).

Anti–T Cell Antibody Treatment

Even with the triad of prednisone, azathioprine, and cyclosporine, many transplant recipients experience episodes of rejection that require additional immunosuppression. Faced with evidence of organ rejection, the initial approach usually is to administer a pulse of high-dose steroids. This treatment may be repeated after one or two days, and about one-third to one-half of acute rejection episodes are reversed in this way. If, however, the steroid pulses do not work, additional treatment is needed. The newest immunosuppressive drugs—and the next treatment alternative—are sophisticated antibody preparations directed specifically at the T cells of the immune system, which mediate the rejection process. These new drugs are the product of modern biotechnology, which holds extraordinary promise for the future of organ transplantation.

OKT3 (Orthoclone)

OKT3 is an antibody. As described earlier, an antibody is a protein produced naturally by the immune system to protect the body from onslaught by foreign invaders. OKT3 is a unique substance in that it binds by contact only to T cells. Its specificity comes from its having an affinity for the antigens that reside on the body's T cells, but not for the antigens associated with other cells of the immune system. OKT3 can thereby temporarily eliminate the exact cells responsible for acute rejection. Indeed, the principal drawback of OKT3 is its extraordinary power to suppress the immune system—so much so that it can be used only for a relatively short time without leaving the transplant recipient literally defenseless against infection. OKT3 is so effective at suppressing the immune system that even a virus that has been residing dormant in the body for years may produce infection during the time of maximal immune suppression by the drug.

Developed during the 1980s, OKT3 is one of a new group of drugs that are called monoclonal antibodies, because they contain only one type of antibody. OKT3 was created by introducing human T cells into a mouse. Challenged by the foreign cells, the mouse's immune system responded by making antibodies specific to the T cells' surface antigens. Actually, the mouse produced many different antibodies, so that researchers had to isolate the OKT3 they felt would be beneficial for medical treatment. In addition, investigators used a newly developed technology to make a *hybridoma*, a fusion of two different cells. With this technique the B cell that made the OKT3 was fused with a cancer cell that has the unique ability to regenerate perpetually under laboratory conditions. In this way, a biological factory to produce OKT3 (the OKT3 hybridoma) was constructed, capable of turning out enormous quantities of OKT3 antibody without contamination by other antibodies.

OKT3 may be given to prevent rejection, but it is most often used to reverse an episode of rejection in progress. To reverse ongoing rejection, it usually is administered intravenously each day for approximately ten to fourteen days. In some instances, even longer treatment may be required. During this time, the T cells disappear virtually entirely from the recipient's immune system. If blood tests indicate that the T cells are returning too quickly, we may administer a higher dose of OKT3. OKT3 treatment is so effective that it reverses rejection in over 90 percent of transplant recipients.

Like other medicines, OKT3 has potentially harmful side-effects. For instance, the first dose actually stimulates T cells to become active. Before the T cells are eliminated, they release chemicals into the bloodstream that often cause a reaction characterized by fever, shaking chills, and wheezing. In addition, some people experience headaches, while others develop diarrhea. Some of these side-effects can often be lessened by giving additional steroids before initiating OKT3 treatment. Antihistamines (Benadryl) and acetaminophen (Tylenol) can be given to reduce the fever. Once the first battery of T cells is eliminated, the later doses of OKT3 generally cause few side-effects. Fortunately, the side-effects of OKT3 are rarely dangerous, and once treatment is stopped the T cells return to the immune system. This is a mixed blessing, however, because in about one-third of recipients the T cells will produce a new acute rejection episode. This will necessitate repeating the treatment, usually starting again with several steroid pulses, followed in some cases by more anti–T cell antibody therapy.

Another problem associated with OKT3 stems from the fact it is produced from mouse cells, and that the human body recognizes the mouse antibodies as a foreign substance. Therefore, a patient's B cells may begin to make antibodies that bind to the mouse OKT3 antibody, and that will block the drug's action. The human antibodies will make it more difficult to use OKT3 a second time, as the immune system will be primed against it. Usually, it is possible to overcome this effect by giving larger doses of OKT3.

In addition to aborting episodes of acute rejection, a new strategy called prophylactic OKT3 uses OKT3 to *prevent* rejection. A few transplant centers employ this approach for all recipients during the first several weeks after transplantation, while others use it only when there appears to be a very high likelihood that a particular recipient will experience rejection. A third method is to use prophylactic OKT3 when the side-effects of other medicines are likely to be especially damaging. One example of this approach is to administer OKT3 when a new kidney is functioning poorly immediately after transplantation because it has been without adequate blood supply for a prolonged period. When this occurs, the toxic effects of cyclosporine on the transplanted kidney may be particularly harmful, so OKT3 is substituted for CsA until the new organ functions appropriately.

ATG (Atgam and others)

Before the technology to produce OKT3 was developed, antibody preparations were created by the injection of human T cells into rabbits, horses, or other animals. Portions of the blood from these animals were then purified and given to transplant recipients to temporarily eliminate their T cells. In principle this treatment is like OKT3 therapy, but with the critical difference that unlike the OKT3 hybridoma, which produces only one type of antibody, the blood of an animal contains many types of antibodies. Most are not directed specifically at T cells, so that much larger quantities of the medicine must be given to accomplish the same anti–T cell effect. These animal preparations have been given different names, including ATG for anti-thymocyte globulin, ALS for anti-lymphocyte serum and ALG for anti-lymphocyte globulin.

Compared to OKT3, one advantage of these preparations is that they contain so many different antibodies that the chance of mounting an immune response against the relatively small number of anti–T cell antibodies is small. Therefore, these preparations can be used on several occasions without fear that their effectiveness will be neutralized. Their main disadvantage is that they must be administered intravenously in very large volumes. Large volumes, in turn, require large veins, with access to the bloodstream either by arteriovenous fistula (a surgical communication made between an artery and a vein) or by intravenous lines inserted into the subclavian vein that runs under the collarbone. With the new biotechnology that makes it possible to manufacture large amounts of easier-to-use OKT3, the demand for ATG and other similar preparations has declined in recent years. They are, therefore, not always available. Nevertheless, ATG or ALS remains another weapon in the fight against organ rejection.

Cyclophosphamide (Cytoxan)

Cytoxan is the trade name for cyclophosphamide, a drug sometimes used instead of azathioprine to maintain immunosuppression. It is also a chemotherapeutic agent often used to treat cancer. It is used in much lower doses, however, in the transplant setting.

Cyclophosphamide is particularly useful when drug side-effects, such as liver dysfunction, preclude using azathioprine. In addition, cyclophosphamide is known to be beneficial in a number of kidney diseases, such as focal glomerulosclerosis. Therefore, a transplant recipient who had one of these conditions in his or her native kidneys will receive cyclophosphamide to reduce the likelihood of developing the problem in the transplanted organ.

The most worrisome side-effect of cyclophosphamide, as of azathioprine, is impairment of bone marrow function. In addition, cyclophosphamide can inflame the urinary bladder, even occasionally causing bloody urinary discharge. Therefore, it should not be taken in the evening when it will remain overnight in the bladder.

Radiation

In the earliest days of organ transplantation, radiation was the first line of attack on organ rejection. Even after the initial experimental period, radiation was used frequently; but with the advent of modern medication-based immunosuppression, it is now used only in one of the following two ways. First, for recipients experiencing severe rejection, the radiation beam can be directed at their transplanted organ. Given over four days in a relatively low dose, the treatment produces no discernible side-effects. A second strategy is to administer radiation to areas of the body that contain large numbers of lymph nodes. This treatment, *total lymphoid irradiation* (TLI), has been effective in certain kinds of cancers, including Hodgkin's disease, a cancer of the lymph glands, and it turns out to be very beneficial in preventing rejection. Prospective transplant recipients receiving TLI are given small doses of radiation almost daily for several weeks, and often undergo surgical removal of the spleen as part of the treatment. Even though the doses of radiation are relatively small, there usually are some side-effects, including nausea, malaise (a general sense of feeling poorly), and low blood cell counts. Sometimes, treatments may have to be interrupted temporarily because of these side-effects, especially if the blood counts drop. There may also be some long-term dangers to TLI which are not yet clearly under-stood.

Because TLI is cumbersome, somewhat unpleasant, and probably somewhat risky, it is generally not used for every transplant candidate. It may be most useful for patients who have already rejected one or several organs, and who therefore seem to need more potent immunosuppression than the av-erage recipient.

Actinomycin D (Dactino)

Actinomycin D is a medicine administered intravenously, which has an effect somewhat like that of radiation in that it relatively nonspecifically suppresses bone marrow function. Thus, the principal side-effect of actinomycin D is reduced blood cell counts, which must therefore be monitored routinely during use of this medication. When employed in the trans-plant setting, actinomycin D appears to be most effective in treating chronic rejection. In these instances, it is given once every four to six weeks. It also seems to be helpful for the relatively few patients who have difficulty decreasing their dose of steroids without the assistance of another medication during the period of transition.

Experimental Treatments

Undeniably, the advances in immunosuppression have, in a very few years, paved the way for significant improvement in organ transplantation. But no one in the field is complacent. Certainly, as long as recipients suffer rejection and drug side-effects, we will continue to search for new and better medi-cations to add to those already described in this chapter.

Two drugs that appear promising are FK506, another cyclic chemical compound distantly related to cyclosporine, and 15-Deoxyspergualin, a derivative of spergualin, a compound originally discovered in 1981 to have anticancer properties. At this point it is too early to know how useful FK506 or 15-Deoxyspergualin will be. Both are powerful, nonspecific immunosuppressive drugs, and when tested in animals, both have been shown to have significant toxic side-effects. It is unlikely that either of these drugs—or any other *nonspecific* immunosuppressive for that matter—will bring about a dramatic new breakthrough in transplantation, since all nonspecific agents share the same major drawback: they reduce the body's defenses against infection. More likely, these new medicines will find their place in a mix of several different drugs chosen to minimize side-effects, while maintaining adequate immunosuppression, for each individual recipient.

Efforts to achieve *specific* immunosuppression are also being tested, and clearly hold the greatest promise for the future of successful organ transplantation. The hope is to develop a way to prevent the body from attacking the replacement organ, while preserving the immune system's vital role in protecting the body from foreign invaders and disease generally. In this regard, new antibody preparations—in effect the improved descendants of OKT3—may be the "magic bullets." One strategy is to develop antibodies directed at surface antigens on cells that represent only a small fraction of all the T cells in the body. In contrast to OKT3, these antibodies would leave most of the body's T cells intact. It is hoped that such a drug would be as effective as OKT3 in preventing rejection, but would cause less nonspecific immunosuppression. Additional monoclonal antibodies are being developed to target the surface antigens of other cells in the immune system. As yet there is no way to predict exactly which avenue of research will be most successful, but it is safe to say that achieving specific immunosuppression would change the field of transplantation dramatically.

4

Infection

Organ transplantation is currently our best way to fully rehabilitate patients with kidney, heart, or liver failure. Every day of the week, throughout the world, and with a success rate of more than 85 percent at the best transplant centers, we are effectively replacing old organs with new. What only a few decades ago was merely a dream now becomes a reality for thousands of seriously ill persons every year. Moreover, in the next few years, it seems fairly certain that even more organs and tissues will be added to the list of those transplanted successfully.

At this time, the two major barriers to successful transplantation are rejection and infection—two processes closely linked because transplant recipients require lifelong immunosuppression. While suppressing the immune system is necessary to prevent organ rejection, it also weakens the body's ability to fight off infection. Fortunately, in recent years, we have learned ways to reduce the risk of rejection while still maintaining adequate defenses against contagious diseases.

The task of preventing infection actually begins before surgery, in accurately typing and matching donor and recipient. Making a good match helps limit the doses of immunosuppressive drugs that must be taken, and lower doses in turn allow better defenses against infection. Medicines, principally antibiotics, are also administered to prevent infection. This kind of therapy is called *prophylaxis*, the medical term for prevention. Used in the immediate postoperative period, and at times when more intensive immunosuppression is needed to prevent or reverse rejection, these drugs provide an extra measure of protection. A vast array of antimicrobial drugs are also available to treat active infections, but generally the best strategy is to avoid such problems. Finally, but certainly not insignificantly, there are relatively simple measures that recipients and their loved ones can take to decrease the risk of contracting a contagious disease. These we will discuss in greater detail throughout this chapter. The important point is that the result of all these strategies is a healthier recipient, a well-functioning transplant, and for most patients, an excellent quality of life.

Reducing the Risks

The risk of acquiring an infection is determined by two factors: the body's state of immunosuppression and its exposure to a potentially infectious agent. The first part of the equation—what we call the *net state of immunosuppression*—is determined by many factors, including the immunosuppressive medications, injury, nutrition, and general health status. A very low white blood cell count (called granulocytopenia), for instance, or an injury (such as a burn), increases the risk of infection. It is important that patients keep as fit as possible, eat well, and get regular exercise. It is also useful to take simple measures, such as wearing gloves while gardening, to avoid injuries in and around the house. Transplant teams, in turn, are scrupulous about caring for the intravenous lines, urinary catheters, chest tubes, and other medical devices that are sometimes required. And, we are exceedingly careful about removing these "foreign bodies" promptly after the operation, and trying to avoid using them whenever possible. This is especially important immediately following transplant surgery, when the body's defenses are down and the immunosuppressive medications are at their maximum level.

The second part of the equation is the *epidemiologic factors,* so named for the branch of medicine concerned with the spread of contagious diseases. While it is important to limit a recipient's contact with potentially infectious organisms, we are also conscious that the world around us is filled with microbes. It is not possible—or desirable—to live in a bubble. On the contrary, the goal is for transplant recipients to have a full life, including the opportunity to work, enjoy recreation, and travel. To accomplish this we suggest reasonable measures that will control exposure to infectious diseases without unduly limiting one's life-style. When exposure occurs, we then suggest adopting a prudent plan to avoid a serious episode: getting additional rest, eating well, and avoiding unnecessary additional exposure to infectious agents. Sometimes it is wise to take prophylactic medications.

Surgery

Mindful of the risks of immunosuppressing drugs, we take measures before surgery to eradicate potential sources of infection. For instance, this may mean removing diseased teeth or performing a clean-up operation to remove a diseased kidney. In addition, a routine part of the workup before surgery includes tests designed to discover a silent infection, such as cultures of urine and blood, a chest X-ray, and a skin test for tuberculosis. It may also be important to examine stool specimens. If an infection is uncovered it will be treated aggressively, sometimes even if this means delaying surgery. In addition to looking for current, active infection, we run blood tests to look for earlier exposure to certain common viruses, such as cytomegalovirus and hepatitis. Prior contact with the virus may confer an important degree of immunity. Often, this information is helpful later when planning immunosuppressive therapy or considering prophylactic measures.

Next, the effort to prevent infection moves to the operating room, where the surgeons perform a technically impeccable procedure. Minimizing the trauma of surgery limits the patient's susceptibility to infection later. During the recovery period, along with being ever mindful about promptly removing all the tubes and devices, we carefully monitor the white blood cell count. In response to these laboratory tests, it is possible to adjust the dose of immunosuppressive medications and thereby to keep up the body's cellular defense network. Further, we take stringent measures to limit the potential exposure to infection, even prohibiting flowers and plants on the Transplant Unit, since they can carry a variety of potentially harmful microorganisms. Finally, to prevent accidental contamination from microorganisms in the air during those periods when immunosuppression is at its maximum, transplant patients are cared for in special rooms that have powerful filters (called HEPA filters) which remove potential pathogens. During such times, relatives and friends are asked not to visit if they may be harboring an infection—even a relatively minor cold. We also ask recent recipients to wear masks when they are being transported around the hospital for X-rays or other procedures. As time passes, and the net state of immunosuppression diminishes, such precautions are not needed and a normal lifestyle is quite possible, and, indeed, is the rule.

An Infection Timetable

Following a transplant, it is useful to divide the times when the recipient is susceptible to infection into three different periods. There is the first month after the transplant, when more than 95 percent of the infections are those that may be seen in anyone recuperating from surgery, such as urinary tract infections, wound infections, and pneumonia. In recent years, with increasing skill and experience on the part of surgical teams, the frequency of these problems has decreased dramatically. The second phase of the timetable occurs roughly between the second and fourth months. During this interval, viral infections are especially common, and we are particularly concerned about cytomegalovirus (CMV), Epstein-Barr virus (EBV, which causes mononucleosis), and hepatitis. These viruses not only cause illness but further depress the immune system, thereby increasing susceptibility to other infections. Common signs of these infections are fever, loss of appetite, and fatigue. At the third stage, after about six months, the transplant is usually working quite well and immunosuppression is at a relatively low level, and as a result most recipients are remarkably free from infection. Moreover, if they catch a cold or the flu, recovery is much like that for anyone else.

Unfortunately, a few recipients—happily their numbers are decreasing all the time—have chronic viral infections that result in damage to a variety of organs and a persistently and undesirably low overall level of immune function. This may occur, for instance, if a patient contracts a case of hepatitis that does not clear fully within two to three months. Not only may such patients have symptoms related to abnormal liver function (like jaundice, nausea, and loss of appetite), but they are likely also to suffer from repeated colds, flu, or other infectious diseases. Some of these infections may be serious and require hospitalization.

Given the importance of these viral infections, there may be times when either antiviral drugs or antibody therapies are prescribed. Although taking these drugs is often inconvenient—for instance, it may require coming to the hospital for intermittent intravenous infusions every week or two during the first few months after transplantation, or taking large numbers of pills daily—they are effective for preventing certain serious infections. Typically, these measures are necessary only for patients at relatively high risk, and the inconveniences turn out to be a rather small price to pay. The emphasis always is on preventing infection rather than relying solely on treating infection.

Urinary Tract Infection

Infections of the urinary tract, and of the replacement kidney itself, have been significant problems for renal transplant recipients. The signs of a urinary infection include one or more of the following:

- Discomfort or pain while urinating.
- Urinating with increased frequency.
- Fever.
- Chills.
- Pain in the flank area.

An infection of the urinary tract can be serious, even life-threatening, if it spreads to the bloodstream. Careful studies performed over the last decade have demonstrated that pro-phylactic doses of drugs such as trimethoprim-sulfamethoxa-zole (Bactrim), trimethoprim, and ciprofloxacin, taken once daily at bedtime, can essentially eliminate this problem. In addition, it is clear that such therapy can help prevent other important forms of infection. For this reason, we routinely prescribe one or more of these medications at various intervals during the first four to twelve months after kidney transplan-tation. The exact choice of drugs depends on individual factors such as allergies, age, and immune function.

Pneumonia

The term pneumonia means inflammation of the lung, which in the transplant recipient virtually always connotes invasion of the lung by a microbe: a virus, bacterium, or fungus. Almost any microorganism is at least theoretically capable of invading the lung, and since the most effective treatment requires know-ing the exact cause, we place great emphasis on making a precise diagnosis—even when this means performing a surgi-cal lung biopsy. For a transplant recipient it is important to act with special promptness, because the impact of an episode of pneumonia depends largely on how quickly effective therapy is begun. In order to be alert for the earliest signs of pneu-monia, we take chest X-rays once or more per week while the recipient is in the hospital. Later, if there is an unexplained fever, or respiratory symptoms like a cough or shortness of breath, follow-up chest X-rays are obtained.

Special Viral Infections

Viral infections in organ transplant recipients can be divided into two general categories. First, there are those infections, like influenza, to which the entire community is susceptible. Second, there are other infections, such as those caused by the herpes and hepatitis viruses and the papovaviruses, to which transplant recipients are at higher-than-average risk.

The first category, perhaps best exemplified by the flu, reminds us that certain viruses circulate rather freely in the general community. Although many people get the flu, a transplant recipient is more susceptible than the average person. And, if he or she gets the flu, it is likely to be more debilitating and take longer to clear. During one recent community-wide epidemic of influenza in Boston, for instance, many organ recipients had to be hospitalized; other people got the flu, of course, but they did not need inpatient care. The following are suggestions regarding the flu and other common community viruses:

- Take reasonable precautions to avoid contact with the respiratory secretions of people with respiratory infections.

- Avoid crowded malls, theaters, and other public places during flu season.

- Wear a face mask at times when the risk of contact with respiratory viruses is high.

- Ask loved ones and friends to refrain from close contact if they think they may be ill.

- Ask your transplant team about preventive strategies—such as a flu shot or the antiviral drug amantadine—during community-wide influenza outbreaks.

Even more important are the infections that can further suppress the immune system. They may produce a serious *superinfection,* so named because it is superimposed on the original viral condition. Potentially caused by a wide variety of microbial agents that do not normally cause infection in the average person, a superinfection can be life-threatening. Moreover, by a mechanism that is different from classical rejection, these viruses may cause injury to the transplanted organ. Additionally, these viruses may participate in a process—not fully understood—that causes relatively rare kinds of cancer.

The most common, and most important, of these infections is caused by the herpes group of viruses, including cytomegalovirus (CMV), Epstein-Barr virus (EBV), herpes simplex virus (HSV), and varicella-zoster virus (VZV). Once a person is infected, these viruses reside in the body in a latent state. This is dangerous for a transplant recipient, because the virus may reactivate at a later date when the body's resistance is low, such as when the immunosuppressive therapy must be increased to prevent or treat rejection. We are especially wary of CMV, because about half the people in the United States have been exposed to this virus. Fortunately, there are relatively simple blood tests to detect exposure, and these are routinely obtained before transfusion or transplantation. Both blood and donor organs are similarly tested for CMV. Three basic strategies for preventing active CMV disease currently under investigation are weekly intravenous administration of anti-CMV hyperimmune globulin, antiviral drugs such as acyclovir (Zovirax) and ganciclovir (Cytovene), and a combination of the two approaches.

We also are concerned about the Epstein-Barr virus, or EBV, not only because it produces a troubling chronic flu-like illness, but because it can also cause a rather uncommon type of cancer known as EBV-related lymphoproliferative disease. Fortunately, this disease has occurred in less than 2 percent of transplant recipients. We are instituting an antiviral treatment program for EBV similar to the one just described for CMV.

In recent years, the press has publicized problems with the

herpes simplex virus (HSV). For organ transplant recipients, HSV produces the same kind of inflammation and ulceration of the mouth, esophagus, genital area, or anus that it does in the general population. While HSV occurs in as many as 40 percent of recipients, HSV infection is readily treated with oral or intravenous acyclovir or with other antiviral drugs.

In the general population, varicella-zoster virus (VZV) can cause chickenpox and zoster (shingles). Chickenpox occurs with the initial or primary infection, while zoster arises when the virus is reactivated—usually well into adulthood. At least 90 percent of transplant recipients have latent VZV, largely due to exposure during childhood. However, only about 10 percent develop zoster, with fever, pain, and a localized rash of blisters on reddish or inflamed skin. Shingles is not a life-threatening condition, and can be treated with over-the-counter remedies to ameliorate the symptoms. More serious episodes can be treated with antiviral drugs. In contrast, VZV infection can be very serious for someone who has never had chickenpox or zoster—a person who is VZV antibody-negative. For this reason, we routinely check a recipient's antibody status before transplantation. Antibody-negative individuals are notified of their status, and are instructed to avoid, as much as possible, contact with the virus. A patient who is exposed to the virus should report this *immediately* to the transplant team so that appropriate preventive measures, such as an antivaricella antibody, can be immediately administered. This point is especially important for children, who are much more likely than adults to come in contact with the chickenpox virus.

In the past, about 10 percent of transplant recipients have contracted chronic hepatitis, due to either the hepatitis B virus or the so-called non-A non-B hepatitis virus(es), nowadays also called hepatitis C. Typically, people became infected at the time of transplantation. However, with better methods for testing both blood and donor organs, this way of contracting the virus is becoming less common. Currently, the majority of recipients who have chronic hepatitis were infected before their transplant surgery. While hepatitis causes several short-term problems related to abnormal liver function, chronic hepatitis combined with long-term immunosuppressive therapy can—over several years to decades—lead to progressive liver damage and occasionally cirrhosis. Additionally, hepatitis B infection increases the risk of developing liver cancer many years later. The hepatitis virus also reduces one's overall resistance to superinfection. At present, we do not have adequate therapies for treating hepatitis in a transplant recipient, although there is a very active research effort in this area. The emphasis is, therefore, on preventing infection by very careful testing of organ and blood donors, and on the patients' part by avoiding illicit drugs, high-risk sexual partners, and travel to areas where hepatitis is common. In addition, there are vaccines to protect people who have not been exposed to the virus.

Papovaviruses are another group of viruses that have a special adverse impact on immunosuppressed individuals, principally because they have the potential to cause cancer. One subgroup of this family of viruses causes the common wart, and people whose immune systems are functioning below par have a higher incidence of warts than the general public. While warts are understandably a cosmetic concern, in response to sun exposure they may also produce a potentially serious form of skin cancer, squamous cell carcinoma. It is therefore advised that transplant recipients, especially those with a fair complexion, avoid sunbathing and tanning salons, and use sunscreens with a high sun protective factor (SPF) when they are exposed to ultraviolet rays. Fortunately, attention to these measures essentially eliminates this problem.

Living a Normal Life

Despite the litany of potential problems with infectious disease that can affect someone living with a transplant, the great majority of recipients eventually return to a normal life-style. They work, have a family, raise children, play a useful role in the community, and enjoy recreation. Nevertheless, infection will always be a concern because of the lifelong need for immunosuppressive medicines. The following is a list of do's and don'ts to help reduce the risk of acquiring a contagious disease.

- **Never decide on your own to change your medication regimen.** This may not only threaten the viability of the transplant but also increase the risk of infection.

- **Do not self-prescribe over-the-counter medications such as vitamins, laxatives, and cold remedies.** Acetominophen (Tylenol) is an acceptable pain remedy, but if it does not bring relief, consult your doctor promptly.

- Preventing infection is far better than treating infection. Thus, antimicrobial drugs are usually prescribed before any kind of invasive diagnostic or therapeutic procedure, from dental work to major surgery. **Inform the transplant team if you anticipate having any invasive procedure, even routine dental cleaning, so preventive measures can be taken.**

- **Keep in close communication with your transplant team about medical matters, even those not related to the transplant.**

- A few times a year, almost everyone—immunosuppressed or not—develops trivial infectious problems such as a cold or diarrhea. **Alert the transplant team if you have any of the following symptoms:**

  - Any fever over 100° F, particularly if accompanied by chills.

  - Cough or diarrhea persisting for more than three days.

  - More than three *hours* of shortness of breath, difficulty or discomfort urinating, abdominal pain, or unexplained headache.

  - Development of a skin rash.

  - Pain on swallowing.

- **Discuss with the transplant team any possible aller-gies, especially to drugs.** They will advise you of whether and when you should avoid these agents.

- You can enjoy travel to interesting areas of the world, but your plans should be tempered by good sense: **avoid places where there may be contami-nated food and water.** In general, travel is safe in North America, Europe, Japan, and Australia. Dis-cuss any plans for traveling to other regions with the transplant team.

- **Avoid intimate contact with anyone who has an ac-tive infection, such as a cold or the flu.** While con-tact with others—children, neighbors, relatives— usually is not a problem, common sense should be used.

- **Contact the transplant team if a medical emergency arises that requires treatment at another hospital or by a physician unfamiliar with your medical history.**

- **Consult your transplant team before any immuniza-tion.** Like the flu and hepatitis vaccines, immuniza-tions generally are not harmful, but they are not as effective in transplant recipients as in non-immuno-suppressed individuals. The tetanus vaccine, how-ever, should be avoided, as it may trigger rejection; if needed, protection against tetanus can be safely and effectively administered with the tetanus immune globulin.

- **Do everything possible to stay in good overall health.** Participate in a regular exercise program, fol-low the dietary program prescribed by the transplant team, and keep your weight in an acceptable range. Perhaps most important of all: stop smoking.

Once stable on relatively low-dose immunosuppression, most recipients not only go back to work but play sports, socialize freely, and even travel abroad. With regard to overseas vacationing, besides avoiding places where the public health and sanitation practices are poor, transplant recipients should be particularly vigilant about the quality of the food they eat and the water they drink. For instance, while food poisoning produces severe diarrhea, fever, and other unpleasant symptoms in the average person, it can be considerably more dangerous for someone taking immunosuppressive medications. However, the precautions we suggest are not life-constricting regulations, but largely involve exercising good common sense. The goal of organ transplantation, after all, is to provide patients with a normal life and good health.

5

Adjusting

When I first saw Joseph Goodman, he was lying comatose in the intensive care unit, suffering from what seemed to be the final moments of liver failure. A severe bout of hepatitis A had destroyed his liver. A respirator was supporting his breathing; IVs were running with blood and dopamine to sustain his blood pressure. The chance of a liver transplant had brought him to our hospital, but he appeared to be near death.

As the psychiatrist with the transplant team, I had come to see Joseph Goodman's wife and sons, hoping to help them with their grief. As I entered the room, one of the sons was calling the funeral home to make the final arrangements.

But soon we were joined by a consulting hepatologist (liver specialist) on the transplant team. He spoke reassuringly with the family about the possibility of transplantation. "I'd like your consent to place his name on the list for a donor liver," he said calmly. Mrs. Goodman and her sons seemed to regard this option with skepticism. I shared their doubt. "Somehow," I thought, "my colleague has lost the proper perspective." I could not recall seeing someone in such a tenuous state undergo transplantation. But the liver specialist found a challenge—and hope—where none appeared evident to me.

Joseph Goodman was put on the emergency list, with the highest priority for a new organ. A donor organ soon became available, and he received the new liver.

By chance, about six months later, I saw Joseph Goodman, as he was striding off an elevator in the ambulatory care center. Appearing younger than his sixty-one years, he gripped my hand in a firm handshake. "Got time for a game of tennis?" he beamed. "My wife and I have been playing, and I've been winning." It was one of the moments when organ transplantation seems miraculous.

The goal of organ transplantation is to enable the patient to live longer, in good enough health to live a meaningful life. The task of the transplant team is to make this gift of life as widely available to medically needy recipients as possible. With the extraordinary advances in transplantation technology over the last thirty years, the principal limiting factors to helping very ill people—like Joseph Goodman—are the availability of organs, the capacity of the intended recipient to meet post-transplant medical requirements, and financial support for the procedure. The psychiatrist's job is to help assess the patient's mental and emotional aspects, to help decide on the best approach for each person we evaluate.

There are, as yet, no fixed psychological guidelines for transplant candidacy. With increasing success of transplantation, we have relaxed our criteria, and make new organs available to people who might previously have been considered ineligible for mental or emotional reasons. For instance, we now accept recovering alcoholics with liver failure and a relatively brief period of established sobriety, as long as there is solid motivation and social support. Several years ago, a woman who was moderately retarded became a kidney recipient, although she depended on the support of an elderly foster parent and a boyfriend who suffered from schizophrenia.

However, in considering what can be accomplished for each patient we must take into consideration his or her social and psychological circumstances. There is little advantage to performing a transplant on someone who is incapable of following a strict regimen of daily medications. In practice, the complexity of the human condition may challenge our ability to choose the best course. But the hope always is to provide meaningful life extension in the face of serious, otherwise fatal illness.

The Evaluation Process

Transplant programs differ widely in how they select candidates. The patient may be evaluated by a psychiatrist, a psychologist, a medical social worker, or by none or all of the above. Some centers use standardized tests of mood, personality, and cognitive function. Others make their decision primarily on the basis of a general impression about a person's health, motivation, and social supports. At our hospital, all candidates for heart, liver, and combined pancreas/kidney transplants are seen by the team psychiatrist for a formal assessment. Supplemental psychological testing is sometimes obtained, and an addictionologist is consulted when there is a significant past history of substance abuse. Kidney transplant candidates are seen with a close family member or friend in a pretransplant family meeting, which is attended by the team psychiatrist, a social worker, a nephrologist (kidney specialist), a surgeon, a tissue-typing specialist, and members of the nursing staff.

The one issue that we are most concerned about in the pretransplant evaluation is *medical compliance*, used here to mean a person's ability to follow the prescribed regimen of postoperative care: making regular clinic visits, taking the proper doses of immunosuppressing drugs, maintaining proper diet, and so on. Unfortunately, there has been relatively little formal study of this issue in the transplant setting, so we often must rely largely on our collective judgment as a team. Among the handful of studies published to date, it appears that the frequency of organ loss due to noncompliance is small, but significant—reportedly between 2 and 5 percent. There appear to be certain risk factors we can pinpoint. In a study we conducted at our hospital, among approximately 400 patients who received new organs between 1983 and 1988, the rate of transplant loss due to noncompliance was six times greater among persons with a history of alcohol or drug abuse that was known to the medical staff. Furthermore, of the five recipients who lost kidneys in this way, all but one were under age thirty-one. Two patients had been suffering from active depressive disorders at the time of their operations. With this experience in mind, when we perform our psychological evaluation, we carefully search for a history of alcohol and drug abuse or depression, especially in young adults. When possible, we attempt to treat the condition and improve their suitability for transplant candidacy.

Elsewhere, the distance the recipient lives from the treatment center and the complexity of the medication regimen (see Chapter 3) have been isolated as factors influencing the success of organ transplantation. These, we can work to modify. For instance, we can work closely with the patient's community physicians to minimize the number of visits the patient must make to our transplant center. Additionally, we endeavor to simplify the postoperative drug regimen, and we actively instruct recipients in properly taking their medicines. We try also to overcome problems related to economics, language, education, culture, and lack of social supports. Clearly, many people with limited financial resources can potentially benefit from a transplant, and it is our wish to make that option available to them.

Even with the best of intentions, medical professionals sometimes make mistakes. Anyone who is rejected for transplantation for psychological or social reasons may wish to consider a second opinion.

Waiting

I was struck immediately by the fact that Jane Wilson, in her mid-forties and suffering from progressive heart disease, might very well die before a new heart could be found to help her. Jane was in Class IV heart failure, which means that she was often short of breath even when resting. She needed help for even minimal household activities, and she seldom could leave her home.

The waiting period was very difficult. Yet it was a time of extraordinary growth for Jane and her family. They had seen their share of tragedy: before Jane became ill, the Wilsons' son died, and their oldest daughter gave birth to a handicapped child. Their younger daughter Ellen, in her teens, had experienced considerable turmoil during Jane's illness. For a while, Ellen was living out of the home and doing poorly in school.

Jane's cardiac illness, and the stressful wait for transplantation, brought on an episode of major depression. Jane had difficulty sleeping. Her appetite declined, and she was sad and often tearful and despairing. She lost interest in almost everything except her children and their needs. With a combination of antidepressant medication and counseling, she overcame her depression, despite continued family stress and her seemingly endless wait for a donor organ. She understood that her high level of pre-formed antibodies or sensitization made the chance of successful heart transplantation remote.

As Jane's illness continued, her daughter Ellen managed to pull things together. In part, I think, she was able to do so because Jane herself was a model of hope and dignity. During one of Jane's hospitalizations, Ellen dropped off some schoolwork for her mother to see and share with us. It was an assignment from her twelfth-grade science class, and her teacher had given her an A+. The work, a series of well-labeled anatomy drawings, was wonderfully comprehensive for any seventeen-year-old, but particularly so for this young woman, who had had so many problems. Ellen began to consider a possible career in a health profession.

Any illness is stressful, but having a serious, potentially fatal illness can feel overwhelming. During the waiting period it is normal—indeed perhaps unavoidable—to be plagued by feelings of uncertainty. Will a replacement organ become available before the next medical crisis? Will the transplant be successful? How will the demands of daily living be manageable? Will my loved ones be able to cope? Will they stand by me? Despite these uncertainties, the story of transplantation is one of survival and regeneration. Patients and their loved ones reveal an impressive ability to adapt to the strain.

When Jane Wilson was readmitted to the hospital with heart failure triggered by an infection, we hoped that a donor organ might finally become available. When she was once again discharged without a new heart, it seemed that life was being unfair to someone who was relatively young and who had paid her dues. Jane had followed through with her care diligently, and had been selflessly available to her family.

"But," Jane Wilson said, "Life is not fair. *Life just is.* Make the best of it."

After waiting for more than two years, Jane did get a new heart. Medical complications in the posttransplant period delayed her recovery, but she persevered in her hope and efforts for a fuller life.

Coping with Uncertainty

The uncertain wait for transplantation is balanced by the possibility that a donor organ will allow for a new beginning. In a study of people on dialysis, those waiting for a new kidney showed overall improvement on standardized psychological tests. Anticipating a new organ seemed to provide hope. This may be even more the case for patients with serious diseases of the heart, lungs, liver, or bone marrow, for whom a transplant is the only hope for survival. Waiting also provides the opportunity to resolve unsettling emotions, such as anger or denial, that commonly arise with a sudden, disabling illness.

The negative side of waiting was evident in a candidate for a heart-lung transplant, who after a year on the list came to the hospital in an acute delusional state. While in the emergency room, she told one of our doctors that she had already received her transplant and had given birth to a healthy baby boy. With a few days of supportive medical and psychological care, she returned to her usual level of coping.

Fortunately, this was an extreme case. However, we have found that many people waiting for a new organ benefit from professional counseling, and all require social support. We encourage transplant candidates and their loved ones to meet transplant recipients and their families, and to attend organized support groups. The camaraderie and altruistic identification frequently help with the adjustment process. One candidate waiting for a heart transplant sent a card to a man he had never met, who was simultaneously in an intensive care unit and on the emergency list for a new heart. The card was a thoughtful gesture of goodwill that appeared to help its sender, who had earlier questioned why someone was ahead of him on the list.

It is helpful also when people can accept that waiting is associated with random events that cannot be controlled. For example, after a protracted downhill course of illness, Edith Floriani was thought to be only a short time from death when she and her daughter traveled to a hospital in another city for a pretransplant evaluation. She required oxygen just to make the three-hour drive. They returned home the same day, only to receive an evening call from the transplant team: "We have a donor." The next day Edith was back at the hospital, and soon she was out of anesthesia with a new heart and lungs. Alive and well eighteen months later, she dances past midnight and is learning to cross-country ski.

Not all of the stress during the waiting period is purely emotional. The woman who believed she had received a transplant and given birth had a chronically low sodium level in her blood. Such chemical abnormalities have significant effects on thought and perception. Severe heart disease may diminish blood flow to the brain, thereby impairing normal thought processes. Chronic liver and kidney diseases can cause toxic waste products to accumulate in the body and eventually to impede normal mental functioning. Kidney failure results in anemia, which also can produce adverse mental and emotional effects.

The psychological problems that arise are thus the result of both emotional stress and declining health. For instance, up to half the people waiting for a liver transplant experience at least some mild impairment of mental functioning, such as finding it hard to concentrate or to remember ordinary events with their usual accuracy. Additionally, there may be neurological problems such as tremor, confusion, numbness and tingling of the hands or feet, poor balance and coordination, or seizures, and these problems may create dependence on family, friends, or colleagues at work. People used to being competent and in control find it emotionally burdensome to feel dependent on others. Patients whose illness is recent are especially stressed, because they have had little time to adjust and develop coping strategies.

The waiting period also can be a very lonely time. Sometimes family and friends withdraw, or are otherwise unable to handle the caregiving tasks or emotional strains. Or the person who is ill pulls back and becomes isolated. We have heard patients with organ failure describe feeling like spectators in their own home. In addition to individual or family counseling, support groups can be helpful. Your transplant center has information about groups in your community, and for further information you can contact the National Association of Patients on Hemodialysis and Transplantation (NAPHT), the Kidney Transplant and Dialysis Association (KTDA), the American Heart Association, or the Liver Foundation.

Others

Inevitably, the most important support comes from the caring of loved ones—usually a spouse, lover, or parent who becomes both coach and partner during the illness. This is so important that "supporting the supporter" is one of the hospital's most meaningful roles. We also encourage family members to participate in support groups.

Unfortunately, the stress of illness and of waiting for an organ transplant is sometimes more than family and friends can cope with. Marriages may break apart, loved ones may pull away. In these instances it is normal to feel great disappointment and loss. Here is what one woman recounted:

> I am divorced now, but was married for six years before I
> got sick. He had been the closest person in my life, but,
> toward the end—before the transplant, when I was very
> ill—he was not able to be with me any longer. In a rather
> abrupt way he walked out. I was devastated. On top of
> the fears about my illness getting worse, I was alone.
> Now, I suppose I can say it was a blessing in disguise,
> because it taught me how to get through it by myself. It
> was a challenge, but I learned to be much stronger and
> that I had the strength to do it.
>
>   Then, there were other people—dear old friends and
> new ones—who rose to the occasion to be part of a loving support circle. Three women friends took turns coming to my home whenever they could—either to be with
> me or to bring me something. Because I was too ill to

cook, they would fix food. I guess you just can't predict who will be there for you, except that you have to be there for yourself.

For the family of a deceased donor, the act of organ donation can help mitigate the loss somewhat. It is currently believed to be ill-advised for recipient and donor families to meet, but at times we have relayed through the organ bank confidential communication, such as this letter from a kidney recipient.

Dear Friend:

I am a forty-two-year-old wife and the mother of two teenage children. There is nothing I can say that will help you to make any sense of your son's death. What I can do is provide some positive reinforcement for your incredibly compassionate and generous donor decision.

As the recipient of a successful kidney transplant, I have trouble articulating my feelings of gratitude and wonder. I literally have been granted a new lease on life, both physically and mentally. I have been transformed from a passive and tired observer of life to an active and vital participant. Not only has the quality of my own life improved immeasurably, but so has that of my family.

The precious gift of a healthy organ is one that I have not and will not ever take for granted, one that gives new meaning to the term life everlasting.

Very sincerely,

A Friend

Anxiety and Depression

When waiting produces dominant symptoms of anxiety, anti-anxiety medications are often helpful. These drugs are relatively short-acting and are easily metabolized (broken down) in the body. Some patients also experience depression, with its debilitating feelings of hopelessness, diminished self-worth, and despair. There are also antidepressant medications, which can be helpful in combination with psychological counseling. These drugs have some potentially serious side-effects, however, especially when normal liver or heart function is impaired. Therefore, they must be taken exactly as prescribed and monitored regularly by the patient's doctor. In addition, many symptoms of depression, such as fatigue, difficulty in sleeping, and lethargy, also accompany failing health. Sometimes it is difficult to separate the symptoms of organ failure from those of emotional problems, which may be superimposed. While many people may commonly feel there is little that can be done for such changes in mood, these symptoms are often responsive to psychiatric treatment. It is important to report such symptoms or troubling feelings, so that steps can be taken to alleviate them.

There are also strategies for coping with anxiety and depression that do not involve medication or psychotherapy. Pastoral guidance, physical exercise, social activities, imaging, self-hypnosis, and a variety of techniques, including meditation and prayer, that promote the relaxation response, can be helpful for dealing with stress. These strategies are virtually free of negative side-effects, and they can improve a patient's overall sense of well-being.

Recovery

Recovering is a *process*, one that takes many weeks to months. Emotional recovering begins the moment one wakes up from anesthesia with the realization that a new, functioning organ is in place. As one patient put it:

> I woke up feeling I had been given a second chance, a second life. I saw it as a transformation. In my last dream before the operation I imagined that I was giving birth. Reflecting on it, I think it was the transplant giving birth to a new me. And that has continued to happen. I feel

like a child, beginning all over again, but with the benefit of my experience and wisdom as an adult.

It is, however, not uncommon for the optimism to change at some point to feelings of nervousness, withdrawal, or even paranoia, particularly if unanticipated complications arise. For reasons not entirely clear as yet, heart recipients often go through a period of hypervigilance in the postoperative period. They often experience anticipatory anxiety before their heart biopsies (see Chapter 7), and they may react with concern to a relatively small break in their customary routines. The team approach to treatment may expose recipients to conflicting information, and this can be unsettling. Whatever the apparent source of a frightening or negative emotion, it is important to bring it to the attention of the transplant team. Emotional support and counseling are an important part of the medical treatment that assists the recovery process.

Shortly after surgery, there may be a time of confusion, particularly while the patient is still in intensive care. One heart transplant recipient imagined our transplant coordinator and Santa Claus were plotting to take over the world. Observing a flurry of activity outside her room, a second heart recipient believed the medical staff was battling over her care. In reality, the staff members were dealing with a medical emergency involving a child in a nearby bed. Contact with familiar people is the best medicine for becoming reoriented during the postoperative period. When it becomes medically feasible, this includes visits from family and loved ones. In addition, a radio, a television, or familiar objects from home may aid reorientation in the postoperative environment.

In this early period of recovery, it is also common to have strong feelings about living with an organ that was once part of another person's body. Some recipients express concern about the age or sex of the donor, wondering if their new organ may change them in some way. One woman, who received a transplant from a young man, described herself as being a "hermaphrodite" and "young again." A former psychiatric consultant at our hospital recounted the story of a kidney recipient who quit the Ku Klux Klan and joined the NAACP after learning his new organ had come from an African-American donor. Some recipients give human qualities, such as a name and personality, to the transplant. One of our liver recipients thought of her new organ as "The little girl I never had." By and large these emotional reactions are transient and can help the patient adapt. In general, we do not regard them as signs of underlying emotional strain or mental illness.

The cohesive nature of the transplant team facilitates the patient's recovery. A common mission sets this interdisciplinary group apart somewhat from the rest of the general hospital. Also, members of different patients' families often get to know one another, following each recipient's progress and providing support. On the negative side, a death or serious complication can be very stressful, even to people outside the patient's family. These events also have a stressful impact on the medical staff.

The bonding that goes on among recipient, family, and the medical staff may raise thorny emotional issues. For example, planning for discharge may seem like being "pushed out the door." Or the team's strict attention to dietary management and medical compliance may sound like criticism. It is important to keep in mind that the medical regimen is designed to maximize recovery and organ survival.

The Emotional Roller Coaster

For most transplant recipients, recovering has its ups and downs, particularly when there are episodes of rejection, infection, or other complications. The psychological setbacks are, of course, partly physiological. Anyone who has had a stiff case of the flu can relate to how it feels to be weak and lethargic. Under these circumstances it is also common to be moody and depressed. Unavoidably, there are links between the immune system and the central nervous system. When the body feels bad, the mind feels bad, too.

Rejection is a common occurrence, and is associated with an emotional roller coaster, as the high of recovery is followed by the low of recurrent organ failure. Rejection brings back the feelings of uncertainty and loss of control that occurred before the transplant. Worries about the potential side-effects of immunosuppressive medications add to the stress, as does the inability of the medical staff to predict the outcome.

During the ups and downs, the best coping strategy is to take things "one day at a time." That means accepting the gift of an organ along with its attendant uncertainties. One can expect it to take three to four months to get through the initial recovery period. Of course, adjusting will be much easier if medical events proceed smoothly than if there are many complications. Overall, we have been both surprised and gratified at the ability of recipients and families to adjust to the stresses of transplantation. Even patients with prior emotional illness typically have exceeded expectations, confirming our belief that *transplantation is a basic course in survival.* Happily, most people benefit from the experience.

Living with Your Transplant

The statistics for overall recovery after organ transplantation are encouraging. Researchers reporting in the *New England Journal of Medicine* in 1988 found that 80 percent of kidney recipients achieved a nearly normal life-style. At the University of California in Los Angeles, investigators report that over 70 percent of liver recipients are working at least part time. The transplant group in Pittsburgh, who have performed the most liver transplants, report that two-thirds of their liver recipients are enjoying a good quality of life. Up to 90 percent of heart recipients report satisfaction with the quality of their lives.

But it is unrealistic to expect that life after transplantation will be the same as life before illness and surgery. There will be limitations. One thirty-six-year-old heart transplant recipient who returned to our center for a third-year evaluation has been free of rejection, but has some abnormal kidney function related to cyclosporine. Another medication, azathioprine, was discontinued when it depressed his body's white blood cells. He is working full time and studying for an MBA degree, and he has been active in recreational pursuits. Often, however, he concerns himself with questions of how long he will survive. And he compares himself to healthy contemporaries who appear to have achieved more in job satisfaction and income. A heart-lung transplant recipient in her twenties complains that she cannot find work that will give her sufficient medical benefits to cover the cost of health care and medications: her cyclosporine costs more than five thousand dollars annually. It is not unusual to struggle with the side-effects of immuno-suppressive medications, or to face the disruption of unantic-ipated hospital care for rejection or infection. One liver recipient has had his new organ for eight months. Early post-operative complication interfered with his ability to work, but he now plans to undertake training for a new career in nursing. A heart-lung transplant recipient who has met with me occa-sionally shows no stigma of her illness and finds each day meaningful and full of creative pursuits. In short, the experi-ence of persons living with a new organ is quite variable, but rarely without its ups and downs.

Drugs: Psychological Side-Effects

In Chapter 3 we discussed immunosuppressive medications, emphasizing their essential role in preventing organ rejection, along with their potential side-effects. These drugs may trigger certain unwanted mental and emotional reactions, which for-tunately are usually dose-related and reversible. In other words, at relatively low doses these medications typically cause few psychological problems, and when problems do arise they are not necessarily permanent. Psychological side-effects most often occur in the early postoperative period, or when rejection episodes requite increased doses of medication.

Moreover, not all of the psychological effects of immuno-suppressive medications are negative. One study conducted at the University of Minnesota found that treatment with pred-nisone and cyclosporine improved post-transplant adjustment, when compared to treatment with prednisone, antilymphocyte globulin, and azathioprine. This is almost certainly because cyclosporine has been so beneficial in producing successful transplant outcomes, and because it reduces the total amount of prednisone needed in the postoperative period.

Cyclosporine

Cyclosporine can produce a number of side-effects that affect emotional well being. One is *sleep disturbances*, such as insom-nia, nightmares, or vivid dreams. Another is *irritability*, includ-ing sudden mood changes. And some people experience decreased memory and concentration. When these side-effects are present, typically there also are physical signs of toxicity, such as tremors (most noticeable in the hands), higher blood pressure, and abnormal kidney function tests. Fortunately, the psychological side-effects usually abate when the dose of med-ication is reduced. Be sure to inform your medical team if you become aware of any new physical symptom, such as shaking hands, mood swings, or difficulty in sleeping.

Cyclosporine has certain potentially serious neurological side-effects, which, thankfully, are not common. As with pred-nisone, CsA increases the risk of seizures. Several researchers have noticed that this side-effect is more common among liver recipients than among other organ recipients. The reason for this is not entirely clear, but may be that liver failure produces its own adverse effects on the brain and the central nervous system. It may be that before transplantation some liver recip-ients already have a degree of injury to the nervous system that predisposes them to seizures. Alternatively, liver trans-plant recipients may have higher brain levels of cyclosporine.

Seizures may occur in a variety of forms. There is the grand mal type, in which the muscles contract in convulsion, con-sciousness is lost, and there may be loss of bowel and bladder control. There are also focal or partial seizures, with uncoordinated movement of a localized area of the body, or complex psychological events such as seeing, hearing, or smelling things that are imagined. Reducing the dose of CsA and prednisone diminishes the risk of repeated seizures. Anticonvulsant medications, such as carbamazepine (Tegretol), phenytoin (Dilantin), or valproic acid (Depakene) are also available to help control seizure activity, but these have the undesirable effect of speeding the body's metabolism of immunosuppressive medication. *Rarely,* recipients have experienced more severe neurological problems with CsA, such as confusion, delirium, or paralysis. It is not yet certain whether these unusual events have indeed been caused by the CsA. As mentioned earlier, it is important to promptly report any new neurological sign or symptom. It may be necessary to adjust your dose of CsA.

It should also be noted that cyclosporine comes from the pharmacy dissolved in olive oil and ethanol (alcohol). Some people taking a medication called metaclopromide (Reglan), and recovering alcoholics treated with disulfuram (Antabuse), have reported reactions, such as dizziness, while taking CsA. In addition, some recovering alcoholics may be concerned about being exposed to the alcohol in the CsA, worrying that it will increase their risk of returning to abusive drinking. In reality, the amount of alcohol in the CsA is too low to be physiologically significant, and has not been associated with relapses of drinking behavior.

Prednisone

In Chapter 3 we also discussed the potential side-effects of prednisone. The unwanted mental and emotional effects of steroids have been well documented since the introduction of these drugs into medicine three decades ago. Like the physiological side-effects, the psychological ones are usually dose-related, so that with the advent of cyclosporine the frequency of these problems has diminished considerably.

Nevertheless, when taking steroids, be alert to:

- Unanticipated mood changes, which may be "up" (euphoric) or "down" (depressive).
- Irritability (often noticed primarily by family and friends).
- Sweating.
- Sleep disturbances (insomnia, vivid dreams, nightmares).
- Difficulty in concentrating.
- Memory lapses.
- Increased appetite.

Mood changes may occur when the steroid dose is reduced or increased. The adverse effects of lowering the dose usually go away in about twenty-four to forty-eight hours, and require no special medical attention. In the pre-cyclosporine era, *steroid psychosis* was occasionally seen, with severe mood changes, altered perception, and impaired judgment. Fortunately, this is now extremely rare, and when it does occur it can be treated with medications.

Body Image

Steroid medications often produce unwanted changes in physical appearance, such as extra body fat (especially in the face, back of the neck, and lower abdomen), unwanted hair growth, and acne. Sometimes patients gain considerable weight. One middle-aged woman who gained fifty pounds experienced poor self-esteem, depression, orthopedic complications, and heart failure, all aggravated by her obesity.

Since we live in an extremely appearance-aware culture, any unwanted physical change can be stressful, especially for teenagers and young adults. It is not unusual for a patient who experiences these effects to be reluctant to follow the prescribed medication regimen. This can be extremely self-defeating and dangerous, since the immunosuppressive medicines are absolutely essential to maintaining the function of the transplanted organ. If you feel like deviating even slightly from the prescribed medication regimen, *first discuss this with the transplant team*. Strategies can often be developed to deal with unwanted hair, skin problems, mood changes, or other troubling side-effects of the medicines. For example, some recipients who have developed common warts, a viral disorder, while on immunosuppressive medications have benefited when their dose of azathioprine was discontinued and replaced with cyclophosphamide. The use of OKT3 (see Chapter 3) for early post-transplant care has allowed some patients to reduce, or even discontinue, prednisone. Another experimental approach, total lymphoid irradiation (see Chapter 3), delivered to the body's lymph nodes before organ transplantation helps to reduce the subsequent requirement for immunosuppressive medications.

Dialysis versus Transplant

Unlike the situation faced by patients with heart, lung, or liver failure, people with severe kidney disease have the option of dialysis for long-term life support. The decision to have a transplant is, therefore, sometimes an elective one, and the issues that must be weighed more often involve quality of life than survival.

In making your choice, it is helpful to consider the experience of others. To date, perhaps the best available comparison of dialysis versus transplantation comes from a collaborative study led by Roger Evans of the Battelle Human Affairs Research Centers, Seattle, which reported that 80 percent of kidney transplant recipients were functioning at nearly normal levels, as compared to 60 percent of those on dialysis. This adds credence to our experience that, for many, transplantation offers an improvement in the quality of life. But transplantation is not necessarily for everyone. Some patients are not medically eligible, and others do well on dialysis for extended periods. Continuing medical advances, such as the availability of synthetic erythropoietin (EPO), which helps avoid the symptoms of anemia from kidney failure, are improving life on dialysis.

In short, as with so many things in medicine, there is no rule as to what is always best, so it is necessary to individualize decisions about health care. Before making up your mind it can be helpful to talk with someone who has had an organ transplant. And, of course, your medical team is available to answer questions and to review the alternatives with you. Stepping back, it is inspiring to remember that only twenty-five years ago kidney failure was almost certainly fatal. Dialysis was still in its infancy, and transplantation a rare event. In an extraordinarily short time we have developed two widely used lifesaving options for people who previously would have died from organ failure.

6

Children

Andrew was a perfectly well child until just after his second birthday. At that point his illness came on quickly, unexpectedly. Mary, Andrew's mother, first noticed that her baby was a bit puffy around the face. She thought maybe he was gaining weight too fast. As time went by, Mary and Lloyd, Andrew's father, thought Andrew's legs were getting puffy, too. They talked about feeding him less, but decided first to see their pediatrician. By the time of their appointment, Andrew's abdomen was bloated; the extra fluid was obvious when the doctor tapped and pressed on the child's belly. Some tests were run. Abnormal amounts of protein were being excreted in the urine. The diagnosis was made: nephrotic syndrome. Mary and Lloyd were shocked, devastated. One day they had a perfectly normal, wonderful baby, then suddenly the sky was falling in on them.

Although Andrew's disease had come on subtly, it was progressing rapidly. He was sent to see a specialist. No specific cause could be given for the problem—we do not know why children develop nephrotic syndrome, which is why we call it a syndrome: a collection of symptoms seen in concert. A course of steroid drugs—an accepted form of treatment—was prescribed. The specialist was guarded, but hopeful.

Unfortunately, Andrew's condition was more serious than for most little boys with nephrotic syndrome. He did not respond to the medications, so after about six months he was sent to the hospital. A kidney biopsy gave an unfavorable prognosis, and another medication was prescribed. This, too, was unsuccessful, so we inserted a catheter into his abdomen and started him on peritoneal dialysis. Now, with his parents, he was making regular trips to the hospital for treatment.

Another six months went by. It was clear he was not growing appropriately. And, while the nephrotic syndrome had quieted down, it was not clearing completely. The final blow was a kidney biopsy that showed his disease progressing.

That entire year was a terrifying nightmare for Mary and Lloyd—shuttling back and forth to the hospital, seeing one treatment after another fail. Now age three and not growing like other children his age, Andrew's best hope was a kidney transplant. A transplant, if successful, would hold out the promise for a nearly normal childhood.

Over the last three decades, enormous progress has been made in transplanting organs in children. Today we provide hope for many children like Andrew who, only a few years ago, would have perished from kidney disease. Progress is also being made for children with heart, liver, and lung diseases. These patients face a shortage of replacement organs, but many of them will receive a new organ, and along with it years of meaningful life extension.

A Child's Special Needs

Periodically, pediatricians find it necessary to remind our medical colleagues what parents know instinctively—that children are not merely small adults but have unique needs when they are ill. Besides lacking the emotional and mental experiences of adults, they are still growing and developing. They require extra time and effort to be loved, fed, guided, and entertained. Their world view is narrower, more immediate, but no less complicated. For our part, we try to provide for these needs when a youngster is ill and must be hospitalized. We realize, too, that needs outside the hospital are vital: school, after-school play, vacation, clubs. We must look to the future, taking on the problem of helping the patient mature from child to adult: advancing education, career, relationships, sexuality, independence. Moreover, all of these factors exist in the context of a family, so they affect parents, siblings, grandparents, each person affected by the changes and stresses of the child's illness. As we remember from our own childhoods, growing up has many difficult moments, and it is reasonable to expect they will be made more difficult by serious illness and transplantation. This makes it important to emphasize how extraordinarily well most children adapt to living with their transplant.

The special needs of children with regard to transplantation begin even before we can consider providing a replacement organ. Under one year of age, a child's immune system is more active than during the adult years. The result is an increased tendency to reject the new organ. For this reason we make every effort to postpone transplantation until after the first year. For children with kidney disease, the option of peritoneal dialysis makes this possible, while infants with severe heart and liver diseases may not be able to wait. In recent years, particularly with the widespread use of cyclosporine, we are increasingly successful in transplanting organs in very young children with life-threatening diseases of the heart, lungs, or liver. Also, cyclosporine makes it possible to use smaller doses of steroids that suppress normal growth (see Chapter 3).

Very young children can be expected to undergo added stress when breastfeeding is interrupted or fluid and formula must be restricted because of their illness. Breast milk provides antibodies that help protect against infections, as well as intimate contact between mother and child, and the infant gains comfort and satisfaction from feeding. So an infant who must stop breastfeeding is likely to go through a cranky period, while the mother too will experience a loss. Fortunately, these feelings pass over time.

Little children also have relatively small blood vessels. And they are physically active. Both factors make it more difficult to perform medical procedures, such as drawing blood, starting IVs, or administering hemodialysis, on children than on adults. While no one likes injections, medical tests, and the like, adults have an easier time understanding why they must suffer through these moments. Young children often do not recognize the potential gains, and become frightened, upset, and tearful. When he was little, Andrew always screamed and cried when it was time to draw blood. We felt bad, but Mary and Lloyd felt even worse.

> As the next year passed, Andrew's growth began to slow, while his kidney function declined. We spoke openly with Mary and Lloyd about what was happening. We began to prepare for the transplant.
>
> Not surprisingly, both parents wished to be considered as donors. They were young and fit. Both went through the medical workup to see if they could be donors. Mary's blood and tissue typing turned out to be the better of the two matches. One sunny, cold day in February, we discussed freely who should be the donor. "Your tissue type is the best match," we told Mary, "but either of you would do just fine." "I want to do it," Mary said without hesitation. We turned to planning for the day of surgery.

Family donors have been used for kidney transplantation since the 1950s, when we relied on organs from identical twins to prevent immunological rejection. A new major breakthrough is to have a family member provide a portion of his or her liver for transplantation. Unfortunately, this is not appropriate for heart or lung transplantation.

There are many emotional issues—some quite difficult—that may arise when a family member considers providing an organ. The most important one, perhaps, is to avoid situations in which a family member feels *pressured* to donate. Since there is a normal tendency to associate the gift of an organ with love, not giving can mistakenly be experienced as rejection— a lack of love. Recently, we had a situation in which a youngster's father had agreed to provide a kidney. The operation was scheduled, but had to be canceled because the child had a cold. As we were rescheduling the procedure, the father backed out. It was devastating for the entire family.

At the time of transplantation, inevitably there is a period of separation for the donor parent and other children in the family. Anticipating this absence, it is important to make arrangements for grandparents, other family members, or close friends to step in and help. Expect, too, that family and friends will worry about the donor, even though these operations rarely produce complications.

As the years go by, children have moments when they feel set apart from their schoolmates by the requirements of their transplant. We tried to schedule Andrew's medications so they could be taken before and after school, but there were times when his doses were increased and he had to make frequent trips to the nurse's office. That meant leaving class for a few minutes, or coming in late. Common viral infections, particularly chickenpox, can be dangerous and even life-threatening. Usually, Andrew was able to play with the other children, but there were periods when he was restricted, and at these times, recess was not fun. Meals were also a problem. Andrew had to restrict his protein intake. While other kids had their bacon and egg breakfasts, he was eating juice, toast, margarine, and jam. The school lunch was often not appropriate; Andrew had to take a bag lunch.

Teenagers generally start feeling embarrassed about their body changes: Am I pretty? Too short? Too fat? The cosmetic changes from earlier renal disease and from the immunosuppressives administered—short stature, acne, unwanted hair— feel like terrible injustices. Andrew was no different. He also resented the periodic medical visits: being examined, wearing a hospital gown. Once Andrew reached puberty, he was particularly self-conscious about being examined by a woman.

The illnesses that require transplantation in youngsters are serious ones that usually affect the entire body. Kidney disease may produce secondary damage to the eyes, ears, bone marrow, liver, or spleen. It reduces overall energy level, diminishes height and body build, impairs performance at school and in sports.

Andrew's first replacement kidney functioned well for about seven years, at which point it started to show some decline in function. At that point he was in fifth grade. We put him back on dialysis. Again, we were concerned about his growth. We brought up the idea of another transplant—at eleven, he still had a lot of growing to do, and although dialysis was now a practical solution, it would make his growth less likely to be normal.

Once more, Lloyd offered to donate a kidney. We repeated the tests and determined that he would be a suitable donor. He was in good health; his kidneys were functioning as well as they had seven years before. So Andrew's dad provided the second transplant.

Now, four years later, the kidney is working well. Andrew is fifteen, back in his normal school routines. He's growing a little slower than his peers, but not all that much. The slower growth is probably due more to the two episodes of kidney failure than to the transplants not doing their job or the continuing immunosuppression. We are exploring the feasibility of growth hormone therapy to normalize his growth rate. The future holds the chances for more normal growth in children with renal failure.

When Mary donated her kidney the first time around, Andrew was too young to understand the emotional issues that were involved. By the time he was eleven, and Lloyd was to

be the donor, Andrew felt both beholden and grateful to his
parents. When Andrew became an adolescent, this was a difficult mixture of emotions. It is not easy to move toward autonomy while still feeling indebted for the gift of an organ.
Mary and Lloyd were quite understanding, watching out for
the tendency to inappropriately use their gift as a way to
control Andrew's teen behavior: making unreasonable demands, raising feelings of guilt or shame, or saying angry
things like "You're not taking care of the organ I gave you!"

Older brothers and sisters may wish to be donors. We are
very sensitive about this, insisting there be no pressure—no
implication that being a loving brother or sister means giving
an organ. We take this problem very seriously, and do not
often suggest that minors act as donors. Minors also have
special protection under the law. A court order is required
before they can donate, and the judge's role is to protect the
interests of the potential donor. It may seem awkward that
parents are subordinated to the legal system in the decision-
making process, but it can be helpful for the family to have a
neutral party involved. It relieves parents of some of the emotional burden of the decision.

Getting Ready

It was a few months between the time we first brought
up the idea of transplantation and the actual day of the
surgery. Before Andrew's first transplant, both Mary and
Lloyd had a number of meetings with the transplant
team, including the psychiatrist and social workers. We
discussed the medical issues and explored their feelings.
There was, of course, far less we could say directly to
Andrew about the upcoming transplant: four-year-olds
do not have an extensive vocabulary. When it was time
to prepare Andrew for the operation, his parents let him
know that an operation was necessary: that he would be
asleep, but they would be with him; that he would be
uncomfortable, but only for a short while. They assured

him the best part was he would feel better and would no longer have to come to the hospital for dialysis. His peritoneal catheter could come out.

Andrew's operation went well. In the first day or two he was up and about. As a result of the transplant, the puffiness went down. The protein stopped pouring out in his urine. "It's marvelous how fast kids bounce back," one of the nurses remarked.

Even very young children need to be prepared for their transplant operation. Usually, we suggest going to the hospital for a trial run. By the time a transplant is considered, most youngsters have already been to the doctor, had frequent clinic visits, and even had some inpatient hospital stays. But they may not have been to the large, often imposing, referral hospital where the transplant will be performed. For any child, from infant to teen, it helps to know what to expect: to become acquainted with the transplant hospital's personnel and routines, the admission process, the hospital room, the procedure. We give toddlers and early-school-age children a coloring book—designed and prepared by the mother of one of our transplant recipients—illustrating what to anticipate. Older children and adolescents get a written list of expectations and services that will be provided. All of this preparation adds up to knowing what to expect, as well as to finding a familiar face when it is time to go in for the operation.

The following is a checklist of items that parents should investigate before the surgery:

- What are the visiting hours for family and friends? When will it be appropriate for visiting to begin after the operation?

- Is there lodging in the hospital or nearby for family members?

- If you are waiting for an organ, but have to be out of town, how will you stay in contact with the transplant coordinator?

- When it is time for the operation, what is the safest and most efficient way to get to the hospital? How soon will you need to be there? What will you need to bring for your child and for yourself?

- What arrangements should be made with family and friends for taking care of the household (babysitters, transportation to and from school, food shopping, meals)?

- What forms will you have to file for your insurance coverage, including hospitalization, outpatient medications, and follow-up care?

For an older child, the waiting period before surgery is very much like that for an adult: filled with uncertainty, anxiety, and difficulty in eating, sleeping, and carrying on with normal routines. (We discuss these issues in Chapter 5.) One quick rule of thumb: parents should expect their child to be experiencing many of the same stresses and emotions that they are. However, the child may not feel comfortable about expressing feelings, so the emotions may come out in inappropriate ways. The child may withdraw: not want to go to school or be with friends, refuse to take medications or go to the doctor. He or she may have problems eating, purposely break from dietary restrictions, or become sloppy in compliance with diet or medications. Or a child may regress and act out: be unusually stubborn, break with toilet training, be inappropriately tearful at times, direct negative behavior onto parents, other family members, or the medical team. Not only is this behavior frustrating and distressing, it also can compromise the medical outcome. But in fact, the child is doing something fairly normal, reacting to uncertainty and loss of autonomy. We suggest two strategies. First, try to talk directly about what the child fears about the upcoming operation: having pain, being embarrassed in the hospital, the transplant not working. Usually there are specific solutions for these concerns that can be addressed by the transplant team. Second, try to shift the focus in the home to nonmedical topics: the place for the family vacation, outings, school, curfew times.

An important issue that is easy to overlook is that in the hospital patients are often subjected to embarrassing—although not necessarily painful—tests and treatments. Children anticipate these occasions and are often anxious about them. Indeed, they may fear being embarrassed more than the potentially dangerous aspects of being hospitalized. Andrew never liked being examined, but especially disliked it on rounds when a number of residents and students would be in the room. One teenage girl refused to get out of bed and walk, because she did not want to be seen carrying a urinary catheter bag. These are normal concerns for children. To deal with them, here are some steps to take before the operation:

- Discuss the operation and hospitalization with the entire family well ahead of time. Encourage everyone in the close family to participate in meetings with the transplant team and support groups.

- Be clear about when you expect to be away from home and who will be taking care of the household.

- Plan a reasonable schedule for family members to make hospital visits.

- Work out a routine of household assignments for everyone. Helping out makes the other children feel they are an important part of the family. But take care not to place too much responsibility or time commitment on siblings, further impinging on their social life.

- Try to work out "respite" times with family and friends, so that you spend a little extra time with the other children and your spouse. Plan family outings.

- Expect and prepare for the down times: complications, restrictions, family conflicts. Make a plan for getting help before things go too far.

Recovering

Most children recover quickly from surgery: the wound heals, they are able to get out of bed, eat, go to the toilet. Recovering also involves getting back emotionally, as well as physically. In Chapter 5, we cover the issues that transplant recipients and families commonly face after the operation. For most, the immediate aftermath is marked by an emotional roller coaster: great highs as well as deep lows. The high comes first: the surgery is over, the symptoms of the disease that prompted the transplant are waning, the steroid drugs are kicking in. Later comes the low: worries over whether the transplant will really work, whether life will return to normal, whether there will be complications. Even for pediatric kidney transplants, which are becoming increasingly routine, these concerns are inevitable. At such times, it is helpful to remember that the majority of children with transplants do quite well—90 percent are living five years or more after receiving their new kidney and two-thirds still have a functioning kidney. The remainder return to dialysis to wait for a second transplant. Sixty percent of children with a new heart and 60 percent with a new liver have good function at twelve months. So the real work, for both recipient and family, is getting back to the task of growing up: school, friends, play, sports, relationships.

> Since Mary was providing the kidney, it was possible to plan the date of surgery in such a way as to optimize the result. So, before the anticipated day, Andrew had two weeks of vigorous dialysis to clear his body of waste products. We tried to be reassuring. "It's become almost routine," we said, perhaps a bit smugly.
>
> It was routine for the first two weeks. Almost immediately, the new kidney was clearing the symptoms of Andrew's nephrotic syndrome: the unwanted fluid and puffiness disappeared, the extra protein stopped flowing into the urine. Then a complication arose. The nephrotic syndrome started coming back: we had to change An-

drew's immunosuppression. Mary and Lloyd were apprehensive. Again, we were reassuring. "We've seen this before," we said. "We know how to fix it."

We began planning for discharge. "Let's talk about the routines at home," we said. "We've got to make arrangements at his preschool, get things scheduled for the follow-up visits, talk about getting him back to a more regular life." Like most parents at this stage after surgery, Mary and Lloyd were not quite ready to have Andrew leave the hospital. "Is it really safe to go home?" they worried to themselves. "What if there's a complication?"

One component of the down time after surgery involves feeling different from the other children, being self-conscious about one's medical needs. While the feeling may not be new, it is something that both parent and child hope will go away with the coming of a new organ. Even the surgical scar is a reminder of being different. Although it loses its pink discoloration in a few months, it remains evidence that one is living with a transplant.

There are also restrictions imposed by taking antirejection medications. Immediately after surgery, visitors and visits have to be limited. Once home, there is an additional recovery period before it is advisable to go back to day care or school, visit crowded malls (especially during flu season), or swim in a public pool. At day care and school, youngsters are exposed to many viruses that, in an immunologically normal child, are just a normal part of growing up (see Chapter 4). Chickenpox, for instance, is a self-limited infection that passes on its own, rarely producing lasting problems. For the child taking immunosuppressive medications, however, chickenpox can be life-threatening. Therefore, early on, and during periods when the immunosuppressive drugs are increased, it is essential to be very careful about contact with anyone who may be ill. Later, when the immunosuppressive medications are reduced, the risk of infection diminishes; a child's life-style becomes much like that of other children.

It is also wise to begin the recovery period expecting that there will be episodes of organ rejection, infection, and other complications. At these moments children naturally feel frustrated and angry, and they not uncommonly take out their feelings on the people who are safest and closest: their parents, other family, or medical caregivers. As in the waiting period before surgery, a child may regress, throw tantrums, refuse to eat. Adolescents often become critical, sulky, antagonistic. There may be conflicts over taking medications, following the necessary dietary restrictions, keeping clinic visits, and curfew. Everyone in the family feels the stresses. The other children may act out, resentful of the time given to their sibling. One family had a problem because one child was fond of eating forbidden foods—like potato chips and fast food hamburgers— in front of his brother who had a transplant. He was angry about the extra attention given to his sibling. In other families, the friction and sibling rivalry come out more overtly—in bickering, name calling, occasionally even physical fights. Parents worry about doing the right thing. At these difficult times, the best coping strategy is to set normal limits for everyone's behavior. Seek outside help when things seem to be getting out of control. Plan to use the transplant team as a resource for support and problem-solving. If things still seem to be getting out of hand, professional family counseling should be sought.

Living

Throughout this book we talk about strategies for coping with the problems that arise in living with a transplant, but it would be incorrect to conclude that most children find life after transplantation overly restricted, difficult, or unsatisfying. One woman treated at our hospital comes to mind. At age twelve, she came to us in renal failure. Her first transplant lasted six and a half years, and then had to be replaced. At thirty-two, she still has that second kidney, along with a college degree, a husband, a career, and two lovely children. One boy with a transplant plays varsity soccer at his high school, two others are on the swim team, a fourth runs middle-distance track. One young man plays left wing on his college hockey team. We worry about his playing a contact sport, but he knows the risks. The point is that a child with a transplant can live a very full life. Transplant recipients can go on to realize their goals at work and in relationships, to build families, to take their full place in their communities.

With all this said, it is important to acknowledge that life will be different for the child living with a replacement organ. First, there are the physical changes produced by the anti-rejection drugs: a round "moon face," weight gain, unwanted hair, acne. These physical side effects of immunosuppressives are emotionally stressful.

> At age sixteen, Cynthia was wrestling with all of the is-sues around attractiveness that worry most girls her age. But Cynthia was living with a kidney transplant. On cy-closporine, she didn't like the way her hair was dark-ened. She complained that the steroids made her "fat and ugly." Little by little, she started reducing her medica-tions, hoping she would have fewer changes in her ap-pearance. She did like her looks better, but she also started to reject her kidney.
>
> We thought she was cheating on her medicines, but Cynthia wouldn't talk about it. She didn't say "I'd rather look normal than have my kidney," but her laboratory tests made us suspicious. We couldn't be certain why she was rejecting her transplant, unless she admitted not tak-ing the medicines. We said there were things we could do to help diminish the changes in her appearance, and we tried to be supportive, including altering the medication regimen to get the doses down. We suggested she go to her beautician to remove some of the unwanted hair and lighten the rest. And we brought up changing her diet, so she would lose weight: eat less sugary and salty foods, less fat, start an exercise program. Unable or unwilling to confront the problem, Cynthia lost the kidney. She had

to go back on dialysis. Just before the kidney was fully rejected she admitted: "I can't bear to look so different. I won't take those drugs. My friends ask me why I'm different and I don't know what to say." Our suspicions were confirmed.

After a while, she began to dislike being on dialysis. So the issue of retransplantation came up. This time we had to iron out the issue that had caused her to lose the first kidney. Now she has had another transplant, and this one is working well. Luckily, she has been able to make it with lower doses of medication, but overall she has had to accept that in some ways her life will be different from the lives of other girls.

Children with transplants must learn to be responsible early in life: to take medicines according to schedule, to understand and recognize potential side-effects, to adapt to periods of illness, to uncertainty, and to dietary and other restrictions. The temptation to feel sorry for oneself, to ignore the routines, is always there. Like adults, youngsters learn their coping strategies gradually, over time. Coping becomes another aspect of growing up.

For children, getting back to school is much like getting back to work for adults. Not only is it essential, but it helps with self-esteem. A stepwise approach to returning to school is generally a good idea. We suggest beginning with a period of home tutoring, which most schools can accommodate. Here are some steps to take before the child returns to regular, full-time classes:

- Have the child visit the school for a day or two to get reacquainted.

- Explore the logistics of getting around the classroom, school, gym, and other activity areas. Make plans to handle possible transportation problems.

- Work out a plan for lunch. For most children, this means taking a lunch, although some school cafeterias can make special arrangements.

- Plan on continuing with tutoring even after the child returns to school, particularly in the first month or two when visits to the clinic for monitoring of organ function and immunosuppression are frequent.

- Make arrangements for the child to participate in after-school clubs, outings, and sports.

- A child who was on an athletic team before the transplant should return to the team in a nonactive role for one to two weeks. He or she should build up conditioning gradually, before getting back to full competition.

The goal of the transplant is to allow the child to move step-by-step toward full integration into school routines and outside activities, whenever possible. Bear in mind, however, that each child recovers at her or his own pace. In sports, for instance, we like to encourage gradually increasing activity—starting with walking and bicycling, then graduating to jogging and swimming, and then to activities like racquet sports and basketball. Initially, it is sensible to restrict weight-lifting, extensive stretching, twisting and turning; emphasis should be on limbering exercises without undue stress at the surgical area for the first four to six weeks after surgery. Extraordinarily, by six to eight weeks most youngsters with a new kidney will have returned to full activity and can be playing competitive sports. Generally, we advise avoiding contact sports such as football, boxing, or wrestling. Certain other sports, like uneven parallel bars, vaulting, springboard and high diving, sky diving, and parachute jumping are also generally not advised. If you can, guide youngsters to more acceptable sports: provide a tennis racquet rather than a football helmet. But don't tell them they can't play!

Club activities, such as the YMCA and religious clubs, help youngsters become healthy adults and part of their community. Dancing, concerts, plays, outings, and trips with other children their age, similarly enrich their experience. We expect that children living with transplants will participate in all of these activities, seeking their full potential as future adults. That is the hope of modern organ transplantation.

Some community activities, like swimming in public pools and participating in large crowd activities, need to be limited. Participation should be tailored to the degree of immunosuppression. Swimming in a public pool increases the risk of acquiring a bacterial or yeast infection. It may be necessary to take preventive (prophylactic) antibiotics during times when the immunosuppression is increased. Avoiding crowds—shopping malls, movie theaters, school events, clubs—may be advised, depending on the time of year and the viruses that are about in the community. During outbreaks of the flu or chickenpox, it may be necessary to restrict some activities. It may also be wise, at times, to restrict travel, particularly to certain countries overseas. Antibiotic cover and prudent dietary habits may be necessary. At times, the normal vaccinations may need to be delayed. Consult with your doctor if there is ever a question.

Transplantation has become an established treatment for organ failure in children. The aim is to replace the diseased organ at a time which allows continued growth and maturation, so that the child will be able to take an active and productive part in his or her community.

7

Heart and Lung Transplantation

Transplanting the Heart

At 5 foot 7, with fair skin, sandy hair, brown eyes, and freckles—surviving on hamburgers, pizza, and Chinese food—Rob Richmond seemed, when we first met him, very much like an average sixteen-year-old. But Rob had progressive heart failure that threatened to end his life within a year.

He was born a healthy child. It was not until about the age of nine that he noticed his heart would sometimes beat in an irregular rhythm. At first, he considered the palpitations in his chest only an irritation. But soon the pattern of strange beats worsened. His mother took him to the hospital. It was there that she recalled an earlier illness, which had seemed little more than a flu virus—with fever and chills, and the usual overall aches and pains that for most youngsters come and go without any lasting ill effects.

Tests in the hospital showed that the virus had infected the heart muscle, producing a disease called cardiomyopathy. Rob's doctors prescribed medicines he could take at home; they hoped his heart disease could be kept in check.

But over the next few years his condition grew worse. The palpitations came more frequently. He tired easily and was short of breath. He could not keep up with his

friends when they played after class. His doctors prescribed higher doses of medication, but his heart still deteriorated, and he was referred to our hospital.

While still hoping we could maintain him on drugs,
we raised the idea of a heart transplant. "We'll try these
medicines," we said, "and give it some time. Maybe his
heart will get stronger. If not, there's still hope for a new
heart." His parents were shocked. Rob just listened.

But his overall health kept deteriorating. His energy
level went downhill. Eventually he could not go to
school, much less keep up with his friends. Off and on,
he had to be hospitalized. We began the tests to see if he
would be a transplant candidate. That was his only hope.

For Rob Richmond, and thousands of other people seriously
ill with cardiac diseases, the possibility of heart transplantation
became a reality in 1967, when a South African surgeon, Christiaan Barnard, placed a new heart in Philip Blaiberg, a fellow
countryman suffering from terminal heart disease. This
achievement captivated the world at a time when most of us
thought that heart replacement was still far in the future, perhaps even an unattainable goal. In the intervening two decades, heart transplantation has provided the gift of life for well
over 10,000 people. In 1988 alone, about 2,500 people received
this new lease on life; each year, more and more patients are
benefiting. The principal barrier to additional transplants is the
availability of replacement hearts.

Our success at transplanting hearts has improved dramatically since Christiaan Barnard's first operation. At the present
time, at least 80 percent of all recipients survive one year
following their transplant, 70 percent are alive at five years,
and 65 percent live ten or more years with a new and well-
functioning replacement heart. As with other organ transplants, our advances are the result of improved surgical technique, greater understanding of the immune system, and new
ways to control the body's normal rejection process.

As it was for young Rob, heart transplantation is only for

people suffering from advanced heart failure or life-threatening disturbances of heart rhythm (arrhythmias) that cannot be treated successfully with drugs or other types of surgery. When we met Rob he had already been on medication for years, and his disability clearly was worsening. Not only would his heart failure continue to disable him and limit his life-style, but it would relatively soon cause his death. Finding him a new heart was an extreme but absolutely necessary measure. Since hearts suitable for transplantation are in terribly short supply relative to the demand, only those in greatest need get them. That means people who are going to die in twelve to eighteen months, and who have a high likelihood of enjoying successful rehabilitation after surgery.

Heart Failure

Most transplant recipients suffer from a failing heart. Cardiac failure of sufficient severity to impair daily activity and threaten life can be due to a variety of causes. Some patients suffer from a condition known as *dilated cardiomyopathy*, in which the heart enlarges (dilates) as the muscle deteriorates and weakens progressively over a period of weeks or years. With its pump function declining, the signs and symptoms of heart failure develop: generalized weakness, easy fatigability, rapid pulse rate, shortness of breath, and swelling of the legs. At first, the difficulty in breathing occurs primarily with exercise, but as the illness advances, air hunger happens even at rest. Because there is not enough blood supply to the brain, there may be periods of forgetfulness.

For others, heart failure is an unfortunate lasting result of an infection, usually caused by a virus, that inflames the heart muscle. The medical term is *myocarditis* (from *myo*, muscle, and *itis*, inflammation). Some patients are fortunate, in that their immune system succeeds in eradicating the inflammation, and over time the failure improves as the myocarditis resolves. For others, like Rob, the heart failure progresses to the point where it prematurely shortens their life span. These patients eventually need cardiac transplantation.

Most commonly in the United States, heart failure is the

product of advanced coronary artery disease and earlier non-fatal heart attacks. Each heart attack, or *myocardial infarction*, creates a small area of scar tissue that replaces functioning heart muscle. Heavy consumption of alcohol, more than two drinks a day over many years, can also cause heart failure. With abstinence there may be improvement, or the illness may continue to progress until a new organ is required.

People who develop heart failure are treated initially with a wide variety of medications. These include diuretics to remove excess fluid, such as furosemide (Lasix), ethacrynic acid (Edecrin), metolazone (Zaroxyln), or bumetanide (Bumex), drugs to increase the strength of the pump's contractions, such as digoxin, and drugs to facilitate the delivery of blood to the body, such as captopril (Capoten), enalapril (Vasotec), lisinopril (Prinivil), or hydralazine (Apresoline). Nevertheless, even with the best medication regimen, heart failure is usually a progressive disease.

Potential recipients usually are referred to transplant centers when a cardiologist finds that their heart function is declining despite increasing medications and modifications in life-style. A key point we wish to emphasize is that the medical evaluation for possible transplantation should be undertaken *before* the illness is too far advanced, since most patients must wait from three to nine months before a suitable donor heart becomes available. We like to see potential recipients for their initial evaluation at least six months or a year before significant trouble is anticipated. By entering people on the waiting list before they are at death's door, we hope to avoid unnecessary deaths—one of the tragedies in our field is seeing people die who could have been helped if a new heart had been found.

Selecting the Recipient

The unfortunate reality is that there currently are many more people who could potentially benefit from a replacement heart than there are organs available for transplantation. The number of patients who have life-threatening heart failure seems to be increasing daily, while the supply of potential donor organs remains small and relatively constant. Not everyone who offers his or her organs for donation will be able to provide a heart that can be used to help another life. And, while we can usually use the kidneys or liver from a donor over fifty years of age, this is generally not acceptable for hearts, because the risk of undetectable coronary artery disease increases with advancing years. Furthermore, one donor usually can provide two kidneys for two separate recipients, but there is only one heart. Suitable donor hearts are thus a very precious resource, and we must have strict standards regarding who gets one. Using criteria agreed upon by the medical and lay communities, we select recipients both for the urgency of their need and for the relatively high likelihood that a transplant will give them long-term survival with a good quality of life. Although many tests are performed during the pretransplant evaluation, the basic principle for selecting a recipient is straightforward: the ideal candidate has severe heart disease with other vital organ systems functioning at or near normal levels. While not every candidate fits this mold, severe and irreversible disease of the lungs, kidneys, brain, or liver typically precludes selection, since significant disease in one or more of these systems increases the risks of undergoing surgery and taking postoperative immunosuppressive drugs.

Over time, the combined experience of various transplant centers has produced the criteria listed below for determining who should be offered the option of heart transplantation. These guidelines not only help us provide our scarce donor hearts to those most likely to enjoy the maximum benefits, but also save seriously ill people from undertaking the physical and emotional stress of major surgery when there is little likelihood of long-term success.

- Heart transplantation generally is limited to recipients under sixty years of age, in large part because young people can look forward to longer potential survival. Additionally, young people usually are better able to tolerate immunosuppressive medicines, especially the side-effects that weaken the skeleton or cause diabetes. When faced with an infection, they tend to tolerate large doses of antibiotics better.

- There can be no evidence of active infection or cancer. Before surgery, steps will be taken to eliminate an active infection or a problem—such as dental disease—that might lead to an infection. A potential recipient who has had cancer must be free of any evidence of cancer for at least five years, since immunosuppressive drugs may accelerate an underlying malignancy.

- There can also be no evidence of extensive disease affecting the arterial circulation to the brain or legs, since significant underlying disease in the major arteries diminishes the chances of long-term survival.

- The respiratory system must be healthy, especially the pressures in the arteries that carry blood to the lungs. Elevated pressure in these vessels can cause rapid heart failure and death of the newly transplanted heart. (As we discuss later in this chapter, a person who is disqualified for heart transplantation because of pulmonary disease may be a candidate for heart-lung transplantation.)

- A potential recipient also must be psychologically suitable, must understand the risks and the requirements for taking medications, and must be committed to participating actively in the rehabilitation process (see Chapter 5).

The Selection Process: Testing

The transplant evaluation involves a few days in the hospital, during which time we perform a number of physical, psychological, and laboratory tests. The cardiac portion of this battery includes cardiac catheterization, which helps us to judge the severity of heart failure, the extent of coronary artery disease that may be present, and the status of the blood pressures within the lungs. A careful search is made for other medical problems such as severe diabetes, active infection, cancer, or damage to the liver, kidneys, or nervous system. Finally, we determine the potential recipient's major blood group (A, O, B, AB), and blood samples are sent to the local organ bank to be available for crossmatching with any potential donor.

We also consider any history of—or tendency to—abuse of drugs, tobacco, or alcohol. These substances can have adverse affects on the cardiovascular system and are particularly dangerous after a heart transplant. We also assess the potential recipient's home and community environment, as recipients need a supportive environment to help during their recovery from surgery, and then over the years while they adapt to living with a replacement heart.

While Rob was in the hospital for his pretransplant evaluation, we talked extensively with him and his parents. He met with our entire team, including the social worker, transplant coordinator, surgeons, cardiologist, and psychiatrist. Even though we had already discussed the transplant during his outpatient visits, we reviewed again the risks and benefits of undergoing the transplant. We made clear what medical and psychological issues he would be likely to encounter while waiting for his new heart, as well as what he could expect from the surgery and recovery period.

The transplant coordinator spent a lot of time going over what it would be like to take immunosuppressive drugs every day for the rest of his life, and how he would have to change his eating habits. "No more hamburgers and milkshakes for lunch," she told him. Rob agreed, even though the sacrifice would not be easy.

At the end of the testing period, it was determined that Rob would be a good candidate for the transplant. "If I need a new heart to be independent again, I want it very much," he said. His mother and father and his brothers and sister were very much behind him.

Waiting

Once the decision is made that a patient is a good candidate for heart transplantation, his or her name is added to the waiting list at the regional organ bank (see Chapter 1). Not every heart is suitable for every recipient. First, hearts must be matched according to the donor's and the recipient's major blood type, so each organ bank lists potential recipients according to their major blood group. Second, donor hearts must be matched to recipient according to body size: smaller persons require relatively small hearts, and larger persons need relatively large hearts. To accomplish this fit, we match by body weight: experience shows that if the donor's and recipient's body weights are within 15 to 20 percent, the new heart will both fit and support the circulatory requirements. Finally, potential recipients are listed according to medical status, so those in most urgent need get the highest priority. Patients stable enough to wait at home are assigned to a lower priority, and within this category they are listed also according to the date when they first enter the registry. On the other hand, people who require ongoing hospitalization because their cardiac conditions are unstable are listed in a category of higher urgency. In particular, patients with advanced heart failure requiring support with intravenous medications or a mechanical device, such as an artificial heart, receive the highest priority, since they are at the highest risk for dying.

Most potential recipients—especially if they live near enough to a medical center to obtain inpatient care when they need it—remain at home while waiting for a new heart. The uncertainty of waiting for a transplant is stressful, frightening, and frustrating. There is no predicting if and when a donor heart will become available, or if the underlying heart failure will worsen. It is an unfortunate fact that some potential recipients—up to 15 or 20 percent in most regions of the country—

die from their heart disease before a suitable donor heart can
be found.

> After his evaluation, Rob was discharged from the hospi-
> tal with a beeper, so we could get in touch with him if a
> heart became available. At first he tried going back to
> school, but he found that he tired easily. He might doze
> off in class, unable to concentrate on the lessons. Uncom-
> fortable about falling behind in his studies, he stopped
> going to school in favor of having a tutor at home. Being
> at home was not something Rob enjoyed—he wanted to
> be with his friends—but his parents felt that keeping up
> with school was the highest priority. The tutor came and
> Rob persevered with his home studies.
>
> "It's hard to tell another kid you need a new heart,"
> Rob once said to a social worker on the transplant team.
> It was difficult to be "normal" with his friends and class-
> mates. At first when he went home from the hospital he
> felt comfortable only with his family. Friends asked to
> come over, but he told his mother he didn't want visi-
> tors. As the days went by, and he felt a bit better, a few
> friends did come to the house. But the waiting period
> was long, tough, and lonely.

In somewhat unusual circumstances during the waiting period for a heart transplant, patients may feel well enough to
continue in school or on the job, but studying or working at a
reduced pace. They carry a beeper or paging device, so we can
reach them any time during the day or night should a heart
become available. Whenever feasible, we like to see them in
the clinic about once a week, to make certain their condition
is not deteriorating. On these visits we ask questions about
general health status, perform a physical exam, and obtain
some basic laboratory studies. There also are periodic sessions
with the transplant team psychiatrist. Counseling helps ease

the strain of waiting for both recipient and family. (This is discussed more fully in Chapter 5.)

Fortunately, the ability to pay is not widely considered as a factor in who will get a new heart. Recently at least one state, Oregon, has passed legislation restricting the use of public funds for organ transplants, wishing to allot the state's scarce health resources for other medical needs. To date, in most states, a recipient's ability to pay is not considered in determining eligibility for a new heart. Nor is it considered relevant for the nationwide organ banking system.

Currently, the average total cost of a heart transplant is approximately $85,000, as compared to the total cost of a coronary artery bypass of $26,000. The cost is slowly going down, while survival is increasing. Nationally, more than 70 percent of heart recipients live five years, or more. In other words, heart transplants *work*, providing years of full life for recipient and family. It is our hope that society will accept the cost of heart transplantation, because it is successful in providing meaningful life extension for people who would otherwise die too soon.

The Donor Heart

Any prospective donor is initially considered for giving all organs possible: heart, lungs, kidneys, liver, pancreas, bones, and corneas (eyes). In general, a donor is considered suitable for giving a heart if, at the time of brain death, he or she was no more than fifty years of age, had no known prior heart disease, and had good cardiac function. Blood pressure and electrocardiogram must be essentially normal, although we can tolerate minor instabilities that occur after brain death, if they can be treated and stabilized before the heart is harvested for transplantation. Clearly, we wish to transplant only absolutely normal, well-functioning organs. Whenever possible, we perform an echocardiogram on the donor heart. This simple sonarlike test provides a picture of the heart valves, heart size, and overall heart function. We find it especially helpful if there is uncertainty regarding the donor's medical history, or concern that an injury to the chest might have occurred.

We also record the donor's weight and blood type, matching this information to the organ bank's registry of potential recipients. The organ bank then contacts the physician in charge of the recipient's care, informing the doctor that a donor heart is potentially available. During the next several hours, additional tests are conducted on the donor, including blood studies to detect infectious diseases such as AIDS and hepatitis. Meanwhile, the donor's family is contacted by a member of the organ bank to give consent for procuring the heart, as well as other organs that might be beneficial to others. Based on the number of organs to be removed, a plan is made for coordinating the operations. Timing is critical, since all the organs of the body depend on the heart. Coordination also involves the transplant recipient, who may or may not live near the transplant center. Since often more than one organ will be transplanted, this means coordinating a number of recipients, transplant teams, and hospitals. All of this becomes increasingly complicated if the recipients are not in the immediate geographic area. Time is the ultimate enemy. Once procured, ideally the heart should be transplanted in less than four hours.

The Operation

Finally, the day came when we heard a heart might be available for Rob. He was at home when we called. "Don't eat or drink for the rest of the day," we told him. "There's an outside chance you'll have your operation today. Stay by the telephone, we'll be back in touch as we know more." Rob was very calm. He said "Fine," hung up, and waited with his mother. Within a couple of hours we were back on the phone. This time his mother answered. "We're fairly sure now that we have a heart for Rob," we said. "It's time for him to come to the hospital. Come to the emergency room. We'll do the blood

tests and chest X-ray, and get things ready for the surgery. Tell him not to eat or drink anything."

Time now speeds up for the transplant team. As soon as
we think a heart is available, we contact the potential recipient
either by telephone or beeper. Meanwhile, learning the location of the donor—in this case a local hospital—we estimate
the travel time required to go to and from the donor hospital.
Carefully predicting the time required for the procurement
surgery and traveling back to our hospital tells us when to
begin operating on the recipient. If more than one organ is to
be obtained, this also means coordinating our work with other
transplant teams. Time is, of course, limited—and precious.
The longer the donor organ remains on ice and preserving
solution, the greater the risk it may be damaged. Further complicating matters are the general health and medical history of
the recipient—if he or she has had prior heart surgery, the
transplant procedure will take longer. Finally, we must also
estimate the time that will be required for the recipient to travel
to the hospital, undergo the necessary pre-operative tests, be
shaved completely from chin to ankles, and have a thorough
shower.

It took Rob less than an hour to get his things together
and get to the hospital. We had called down to the emergency room and told them he was on the way. The team
anesthesiologist came to review with Rob and his parents
what to expect in the operating room. He ordered some
sedatives to help Rob relax while the preparations proceeded. The surgical director of the transplant team
stopped by to see Rob before leaving to harvest the donor heart. And the transplant team's cardiologist came by
to examine Rob and help prepare him for surgery.
  Once the tests in the ER were completed, Rob was
wheeled up to the surgical floor, where the nursing staff

began the pre-operative "prep": shaving Rob from toes to chin, painting the skin with an antiseptic solution, and inserting intravenous lines.

Now Rob, his family, and the transplant team faced the anxiety of waiting and wondering how the procurement operation was coming along. At any time, something could go wrong at the donor hospital, and Rob's surgery would have to be called off. Waiting is always trying and frightening. Rob had his family with him to ease the strain, and handled the situation quite well.

Approximately two hours before the donor heart arrives, the transplant recipient goes to the operating room. There we carefully ready for surgery the skin on the chest, abdomen, and upper legs. Catheters for administering fluids and anesthetic medications are inserted into the arm veins, a separate catheter for monitoring blood pressure is placed into an artery, and leads for the EKG monitor are strapped to the arms and legs and pasted to the chest. When patients are anesthetized for surgery, the sleep that results is very deep. Under these conditions breathing is not spontaneous. For this reason, after the patient is anesthetized a soft plastic tube is inserted into the windpipe. During and after the operation the tube is connected to a breathing machine, called a respirator or ventilator, which mechanically performs the patient's breathing. Administering the anesthesia is a particularly delicate matter, because it can easily irritate or depress an already malfunctioning heart. The anesthesiologist thus must be very skillful at maintaining stable heart function until the new heart arrives and can be surgically implanted.

The two operations—on donor and recipient—are now coordinated very carefully. While working in the operating room, surgeons at the donor hospital conduct a conversation with the transplant team at the receiving institution. Based on their progress and the anticipated travel time, surgery begins on the recipient. First, sterile drapes are applied around the operative field, and an incision is made in the skin to expose the front of the breastbone (the sternum). Using a special saw, the breastbone is then divided down the middle. If the recipient has had prior heart surgery—not uncommon in heart transplants—this can be a delicate matter. The diseased heart almost always is markedly enlarged, sometimes adhering to the back of the breastbone. Great care must be taken while cutting into the breastbone so the saw does not inadvertently injure or even perforate the heart. We then expose the heart and the blood vessels leading to and from the heart. Heparin, a powerful anticoagulant medication, is injected, so that the circulating blood will not clot and clog in the heart-lung machine. This extraordinary machine must now support the recipient's entire circulatory system until the new heart will do the job. Several connections are required for the heart-lung machine to function properly. Two tubes placed into the right side of the heart collect "blue" (unoxygenated) blood from the venous circulation; a third tube placed in the aorta transports "red" (oxygenated) blood from the heart-lung machine back into the patient's arterial circulation. During the operation the heart-lung machine thus temporarily assumes the work of both heart and lungs.

Meanwhile another delicate operation is proceeding at the donor hospital. The blood vessels leading to and from the heart are clamped. A solution that arrests, cools, and protects the heart from injury is quickly pumped into the aorta. With continued care and dispatch, we remove the donor heart and place it in a bag containing ice and a special preserving salt solution. Very sensitive to oxygen deprivation during the time it is not beating, the heart must now remain as cold as possible, preferably just above the freezing point. Clearly, the success of the transplant will depend on protecting the replacement organ from injury during the harvesting process, including during transport to the recipient's hospital. Even with the greatest care, we only have up to four hours to safely harvest the heart, transport it, and reestablish its circulation. And so, even with helicopter and jet transport, that means traveling no more than 1,000 to 1,500 miles from donor to recipient hospital.

Assisted by a resident surgeon and a scrub nurse, the team's surgical director performed the procurement at the donor hospital. Meanwhile, another surgical member of the team was available for Rob at our hospital. The two groups stayed in touch by phone. On this occasion, only the heart was being donated, so it took only a relatively few minutes to make the incision in the breastbone, open the chest, inspect the heart, and begin the careful process of removing it from the chest. While ensuring that life-sustaining blood flow would not be interrupted, the harvesting surgeon clamped each vessel supplying blood to the still-beating organ, dissected the surrounding tissue and vessels, liberated the still-pink muscle, and then placed it on ice in the preserving solution. Then, in a gray and lifeless state of suspended animation, the donor heart was lifted from the operating table and gingerly placed into an ordinary picnic cooler. With both utmost care and dispatch—and without ever leaving the sight and possession of the harvesting team—the heart was rushed to the hospital where Rob, asleep with a sedative, was waiting.

If the timing is right, the recipient is ready to go on the heart-lung machine as soon as the new heart arrives at the hospital. The heart-lung machine is started; using its built-in heat exchanger, we lower the patient's body temperature to 78° F to help protect vital organs during this period. First we carefully remove the diseased heart, taking great care to leave enough of the patient's own blood vessels to connect the new heart. Once the old heart is freed from the chest, the new heart is removed from the sterile, cold container, and brought into the surgical field. It is now carefully inspected, and size adjustments are made to the places where it will be connected to the recipient's circulatory system. Now it is time to place the new heart in the chest and begin suturing. First the two atria, the small upper chambers of the heart, are sewn together. Next, the two arteries leading out of the heart are connected.

That means tailoring to size and sewing the ends of the pulmonary artery, followed by the aorta. Great care is taken to ensure that all air bubbles are removed from the heart and that blood is circulating freely. Once circulation is established, the new heart begins to "wake up" and contract. Although the entire operation usually lasts four to five hours, it takes only an hour or so to sew in the new heart.

Nearing the final stages of the operation, we begin the rewarming process. Using a heat-exchange device in the heart-lung machine, we restore normal body temperature to the recipient, who still is being "chilled" at 78° F. Occasionally, the new heart requires up to an hour of rest on the heart-lung machine while it recovers from its state of suspended animation and reestablishes its own blood flow. In instances where the heart had been arrested for a considerable period of time— five or six hours—it may take even longer to recover.

Removing the old, diseased heart also requires severing its links to the nervous system, which for technical reasons cannot be reconnected to the donor heart. Lacking input from the nervous system, the now-beating replacement organ may require medications to speed the pulse rate. Sometimes we insert a temporary pacemaker, which keeps up an appropriate pulse both in the operating room and for a day or two following surgery. This is a normal occurrence and does not imply that the transplanted heart is not functioning properly.

After the heart has recovered and is beating well, the patient is gradually weaned from the heart-lung machine, and the new heart takes over the entire job of supplying oxygenated blood to the tissues. Once the heart-lung machine's connections are removed and the heparin anticoagulant is reversed, the remainder of the operation is very much like any open heart surgery. Drainage tubes are placed inside the chest, the cut halves of the breastbone are sutured together with five or six stainless steel wires, and the soft tissues and skin are sewn together with absorbable thread that will dissolve naturally in the weeks following the operation. Moving from the operating room to the intensive care unit while still deeply asleep from the anesthesia, the new heart recipient is attached to a bedside breathing machine called a ventilator. Artificial breathing continues until breathing is spontaneous and effective, at which time we begin weaning from ventilator support. The breathing tube—inserted into the windpipe after the start of anesthesia—usually comes out within twenty-four hours following surgery. Since it is impossible to speak with the breathing tube in place, its removal is a source of great relief to the patient.

Recovering

By the time Rob's new heart was delivered to the operating room, the bypass machine was oxygenating his bloodstream. Since Rob had not had a prior operation, his diseased heart was removed easily, and the entire transplant operation took only a few hours. After surgery, he was transferred up to intensive care.

For the next twelve or fourteen hours he was still so sleepy from the anesthesia that he didn't know where he was, or that he now had a new heart. Before the operation, we had told him he might feel as if he lost the day of the operation. Now, when he woke up, he found himself hooked up to a number of intravenous lines, a heart monitor, a catheter collecting his urine, tubes in his chest, and another tube connecting his windpipe to a ventilator.

For the most part this meant that Rob was rather unrecognizable to his family, although they could see him through the glass window separating his isolation room from the hall. Even with all the tubes and monitoring equipment, they could tell he was alive and well. For the first day after the operation his parents could thus view Rob, but not touch him. We like to keep new heart recipients in isolation for the initial twenty-four hours to protect them from potential infection. There is an intercom that goes into the room, so the Richmonds could talk to Rob, but he couldn't respond because of the plastic breathing tube in his throat.

The next day, Mr. and Mrs. Richmond were allowed into the intensive care unit to visit their son. Donning a surgical gown and mask, gloves, and booties, they stepped into his room. Their first words were, "Can we touch him?" "Yes, go ahead and touch him," we said.

The next day, the breathing tube was out. They could talk, as well as touch. The intravenous lines were still in place, but Rob was clearly on the way to recovery. Over the next few days, the rest of the family began to visit. First his brothers and sister, then aunts, uncles, and cousins.

Like most patients, before surgery Rob worried about the pain he would feel after having a major chest operation. We told him that the sensation around the incision would be like having very sore and achy muscles. For the first few days, Rob was so pleased to have a new heart that he hardly said anything about pain, but we gave him pain medications just in case. Like pretty much everyone who has had a heart transplant, he was on an emotional high. And on top of these feelings, Rob began taking the immunosuppressive drug prednisone, which added to his feeling of euphoria.

After transplantation, most people stay in intensive care for five to ten days, during which time life starts to return to normal. Within two to three days, all drainage tubes and monitoring catheters can be removed. Some of the best moments come when it is possible to eat again and get out of bed. The immunosuppressive medications must be adjusted. Once eating resumes, the prednisone, azathioprine, and cyclosporine can be taken each day by mouth.

When all the drains and tubes come out, it is time to get out of bed and walk around. Patients begin exercising on stationary bicycles some time between four and seven days after surgery. It is essential to improve one's stamina before going home. Exercise also helps reduce pain and get the digestive system moving.

Initially, we administer fairly high doses of immunosuppressive medications, particularly the prednisone. As with any type of transplantation, organ rejection is a continual worry. For heart transplants—in contrast to kidney transplants, let us say—virtually no significant level of diminished organ function can be tolerated. If severe rejection occurs in a transplanted kidney, we can temporarily provide adequate support with dialysis, and newly transplanted kidney recipients can even remain stable for a few days without any kidney function at all. New heart recipients obviously do not enjoy that leeway. Their heart function must not falter for even a few minutes. Therefore, high-dose antirejection drugs coupled with intensive surveillance to detect early rejection are the most important part of our postoperative management. If things go well— and they do for most recipients—over the first two weeks after transplantation we gradually taper down the doses. During this time, the monitoring lines and catheters must be carefully watched as potential sites of infection. We administer protective antibiotics until the last monitoring line and catheter are removed. To detect a potentially incubating infection early, we send regular specimens of sputum, urine, and fluid from the surgical site to the bacteriology laboratory. Likewise, we perform frequent chest X-rays to check for evidence of pneumonia or fluid building up in the lungs.

Heart Biopsy
The risk of organ rejection is greatest during the first several months after surgery. Because rejection can create sudden instability in heart rhythm or blood pressure, it is imperative that we detect it at the earliest possible moment. In order to do this, we depend on routine heart biopsies. While research continues into less invasive ways to accomplish the task, the cardiac biopsy remains the standard against which all other methods of surveillance must be compared. At this time, routine biopsies remain an essential part of postoperative care, providing an early warning system for the health of the new transplant. There are two reasons why heart transplant recip-

ients undergo far more biopsies than liver or kidney recipients. First, there are no noninvasive or simple blood tests (such as the blood bilirubin value for a liver recipient, or the blood creatinine value for a kidney recipient) that will identify when the transplanted heart is undergoing rejection. More important, the vast majority of heart transplant recipients have few, if any, physical symptoms during the early period of mild or moderate rejection. Since advanced rejection is dangerous and difficult to treat, surveillance biopsies are thus mandatory. We usually perform them weekly during the first month after transplantation, and then once every two to three weeks over the next eight weeks. If there is no evidence of rejection, or perhaps just minimal rejection, we can then decrease the frequency of biopsies to once every one to two months.

Rob was already familiar with cardiac biopsy, having undergone the test when he had cardiomyopathy. Patients rather quickly get used to the process, which takes only a few minutes in the catheterization lab during an outpatient visit. Using a special device called a *bioptome*, a catheter equipped with tiny forceps is inserted into a large vein, most frequently the jugular vein on the right side of the neck. The catheter is then advanced into the right ventricle of the heart, and three to six tiny pieces of tissue are obtained for laboratory analysis. Each sample is about two millimeters in diameter, about the size of a pencil point. Done under a local anesthetic, like that used in dentistry, the procedure is essentially painless, since the heart lacks nerve endings capable of sensing pain. Facilitated by X-ray fluoroscopy, which allows us to see and guide the course of the catheter from beginning to end, the test typically takes twenty to thirty minutes. After it is over, a small bandage is put over the skin, a chest X-ray is taken, and it is time to go home. The removal of the tiny biopsy specimens is safe and has no adverse effect on heart function. Within twenty-four hours, our transplant cardiologist and pathologist analyze the specimens under the microscope and have an idea if rejection is occurring.

The evaluation of rejection on a biopsy, however, is not a

simple matter of yes or no. Rather, there are varying degrees of rejection, ranging from very mild to very severe. During mild rejection one sees under the microscope a scattering of inflammatory cells, called lymphocytes, interspersed among the normal heart muscle cells (myocytes). With moderate rejection the number of inflammatory cells and associated injury to the heart muscle increases. During severe rejection there is an even larger number of inflammatory cells, along with more extensive destruction of heart muscle. During severe rejection we may also see under the microscope hemorrhage and accumulated fluid in the spaces between the myocytes.

In general, we are pleased when the biopsy shows little or no rejection. Very mild rejection is acceptable, since it is not dangerous in itself and does not portend compromise of heart function. Deciding when to treat requires balancing the need to control the rejection process against the many risks and side-effects of additional doses of immunosuppressive medications; we will accept a very mild degree of rejection on biopsy, providing the recipient is feeling and doing well. Somewhat paradoxically, we may be concerned if the biopsies are always completely "clean," showing no evidence whatsoever of rejection, since this may mean the recipient is too heavily immunosuppressed.

Recovery, Rehabilitation, and Discharge

Within one week, provided their initial biopsy shows little or no rejection, new heart recipients are ready to leave the intensive care unit for a regular hospital room—usually in a unit dedicated completely to transplant patients. It is now time to begin active rehabilitation. Since most transplant recipients were mortally ill before surgery, they usually begin the rehabilitation process in a generally weakened state—underweight and having lost much of their normal strength. An essential part of the recovery process, therefore, involves rebuilding the muscles of the arms, legs, and chest. Work now starts on the stationary bicycle, followed by gradually increasing aerobic workout sessions.

During the second and third hospital weeks, the doses of immunosuppressive medications, particularly the prednisone, are gradually reduced. Before discharge, if possible, we like to get them to a level that will be safe for the long term. We also devote a great deal of effort to teaching patients and their families about the medications, including their side-effects and proper dosages.

> In only a few days Rob began eating. This is the honeymoon time for heart transplant recipients, who now can eat almost anything. We are lenient with their diet at this point, since when they were ill most people found it difficult to take in adequate nutrition. After surgery we want muscle tone and strength to build steadily and fairly rapidly, so the diet is fairly unrestricted and generous. As the recipients get stronger, and we see them do more and feel better, we begin to tighten the reins. Soon, it will have to be low cholesterol, few concentrated sweets, low salt. For Rob that meant limiting some of his favorites—pizza, Chinese food, and hamburgers.

For the majority of new heart recipients, the entire hospital stay lasts about three weeks. Barring a serious postoperative complication—now fortunately a relatively uncommon occurrence—the time to discharge is determined by the degree of disability prior to surgery and the appearance of rejection. Soon after transplantation, most people experience at least one, and sometimes two, episodes of mild to moderate rejection; only about half have no rejection at this point. We expect that the majority of recipients will have an episode within ninety days of leaving the hospital. Clearly, significant problems with rejection delay going home.

Monitoring Rejection at Home

At first, rejection usually displays no physical symptoms, but rather is found on a routine surveillance biopsy. Sometimes, however, rejection appears as a subtle change in one's general sense of well-being, such as an unexplained low-grade fever (99–100° F) or generalized fatigue. Less commonly, the symptoms are more pronounced: the heart becomes electrically irritable with premature or rapid beats or periods of erratic heart rhythm; or the heart rate may slow and contractions weaken, producing fluid retention, weight gain, and shortness of breath during activity. It is important that the patient report any new symptom to the transplant team, so it can be investigated.

The first episode of moderate or severe rejection is usually treated with an added short course of high-dose steroid drugs, known as a steroid pulse, generally given over three consecutive days. One week later we perform another biopsy to determine if the treatment has been effective. If moderate rejection is still present, or worsens, following the pulse, or if after a short time significant rejection returns, we then must add other potent immunosuppressive medications. Right now our first choice is usually OKT3 (see Chapter 3). Although highly effective in reversing rejection, OKT3 (Orthoclone) requires ten to fourteen days of daily intravenous administration in the hospital. One week after the completion of a course of OKT3, another biopsy is obtained, again looking to confirm that rejection has been brought under control. At this point, depending on the biopsy results and blood tests, we may also adjust the cyclosporine dose upward. Other drugs such as anti-thymocyte globulin (ATG) may also be needed to treat difficult rejection episodes (see Chapter 3). Fortunately, with the potent immunosuppressive drugs available today, only a very small percentage—now less than 5 percent of recipients—have uncontrollable rejection requiring retransplantation.

Adjusting at Home

Going home after a transplant usually is a joyous, emotion-filled occasion, but it is often accompanied by a significant level of anxiety, or even mild depression, for the first few weeks. For both recipient and family, it takes a while to adjust to the new way of life. Like most new things in life, adjusting to living with a new heart is a learning process that occurs over time. Our experience is that most people cope better if they are active, especially if they make concerted efforts to continue the long process of physical rehabilitation. Physical activity is stimulating to the spirits, as well as to the body.

Most heart recipients go home about four weeks after surgery, so the vast majority of the subsequent care is accomplished on an outpatient basis. During the first month after discharge, we generally like to see the new recipient twice weekly; then, if all goes well, at weekly intervals over the next month. These relatively frequent visits are needed because the greatest risk of rejection occurs during the first six months following transplantation. This is also the period when other potential complications, especially infection, may arise. We tailor the frequency of visits to each recipient's progress, general health, and overall well-being—for someone who is feeling well, tolerating the medications, and appearing to have little or no rejection, weekly visits soon become adequate. Others, having a more difficult course, may require twice-weekly or sometimes even daily assessment. As the months pass, outpatient visits become less frequent, decreasing to every one to two months for the remainder of the first year. After the first three or four months of visits to the transplant clinic, we encourage each new recipient to return to the care of his or her community cardiologist, who will take up the task of routine, long-term medical management.

Outpatient Care

During each outpatient visit we perform a variety of tests and evaluations. Perhaps most important is the time we take to talk—learning how life is proceeding on a daily basis. This careful history of events, along with a complete physical examination, gives the early warning signs of rejection, infection, or drug side-effects. Whenever possible, we like to chat with both recipient and family, getting the general picture of the rehabilitation program. We also review the medication schedule and doses. Close attention is also paid to any low-grade fever, cough, chills, skin rash, or other symptoms that might suggest a viral or bacterial infection. And we look for any suggestion of excessive fatigue, palpitations, rapid weight gain, ankle edema (swelling), or shortness of breath—symptoms that might indicate early rejection. After taking the history, we usually perform the physical examination, focusing on any signs of potential cardiac problems. Blood pressure, pulse, weight, and temperature are checked. Next, we routinely perform some basic laboratory studies, beginning with a check of the red and white blood cell counts, assessment of blood sugar, potassium, kidney and liver function. A cyclosporine level will also be checked to ensure that an adequate amount of the drug—a therapeutic level—is present in the bloodstream. Frequently a chest X-ray and an electrocardiogram are also obtained, particularly if this is a visit during the early months after surgery. As the months pass uneventfully, it becomes less and less important to do all these tests on every visit.

As mentioned earlier, the other major diagnostic test that will be performed is the heart biopsy. Until we find another method, surveillance biopsies to detect rejection must continue throughout the transplant recipient's life. After the first six months go by without untoward symptoms, we can do the cardiac biopsy less often. Individuals with ongoing or recently treated rejection must generally be biopsied relatively frequently, while those with no rejection may require biopsy only three to four times per year after the first year after transplantation. When a biopsy is performed by a community cardiologist, we like to have the specimens sent to our laboratory so that the test can be interpreted by a cardiac pathologist who is familiar with the recipient's previous biopsy results.

In addition to these routine studies, we ask each transplant recipient to have a short stay in the hospital annually in order to undergo a cardiac catheterization. We perform this study to detect possible narrowing of one or more coronary arteries. Unfortunately, rejection is not confined entirely to the heart muscle. Within five years of surgery 20 to 25 percent of recipients also experience mild narrowing of the arteries supplying blood to the heart; this narrowing is thought to be due to the rejection process. Fortunately, the majority of recipients do not develop this problem in the short term, but concern about this issue is increasing, as we now are seeing recipients living healthy and active lives ten or more years after heart transplantation. Since the replacement heart does not have nerve fibers capable of sensing pain, even severe narrowing of the coronary arteries will not cause the chest discomfort that sometimes warns of an impending heart attack. For this reason, it is essential that we perform a yearly catheterization to assess the health of the coronary arteries.

Living with a Heart Transplant

After a few weeks, Rob was back at school, trying to do pretty much everything, as normally as possible. It wasn't easy for his friends at first. They were nervous when they played basketball and touch football. "They worry that something might happen," he recounted. "They don't trust that it's safe for me to play ball with my new heart."

Rob doesn't talk much about feeling different from other youngsters, or about the future of living with a transplant. He never says he worries about his life being time-limited, even though in some respects it is. But of course everyone's life is time-limited.

In light of the progress we are making with immunosuppressives and other drugs, no one can fully predict what will happen to Rob and other heart transplant recipients. So far, Rob has felt well and has had few episodes of rejection. If he is going to exercise, he warms up slowly, knowing that his transplanted heart doesn't have the same nervous stimulation to provide quick bursts of rapid beats that the rest of us have. Instead, Rob's heart relies on the secretion of adrenaline and other naturally produced hormones to increase his pulse rate. But still he's out there playing with his friends, who have become used to the idea.

The task of cardiac surgery—and heart transplantation is no exception—is to give a previously ill person a chance for a long, healthy, *active,* and normal life. We expect that years after the operation the transplant recipient will look, live, and feel pretty much like anyone else. For example, one of our recipients and his wife are expecting their second child, conceived after transplantation.

Initially, rehabilitation means gradually getting back to being independent in the usual activities of daily living: eating, bathing, toileting, and so on. To accomplish this goal, we encourage a regular program of walking and stationary bicycling; first to prevent further deconditioning, and later to build strength and endurance. Routine exercise testing every six months in the cardiac laboratory helps evaluate the recipient's improvement. For most recipients, it is not long before they can return to almost any form of physical exercise. We know heart transplant recipients of various ages who swim, play handball, jog, and even ski. Generally, if one enjoyed a particular activity before the onset of cardiac disease, one should be able to return to it afterward.

Attention should also be directed to known coronary risk factors: maintaining normal body weight, blood pressure, and cholesterol. We like to monitor total cholesterol several times a year, with the goal of keeping the level below 200 mg%. This figure is the healthy guideline for the population generally. Smoking is, of course, *forbidden!* Smoking—and that includes cigars and pipes, as well cigarettes—increases the chance of acquiring a lung infection, which can be fatal. And tobacco is a significant risk factor for heart disease, as well.

> Over the months after discharge, Rob did well with his diet. He maintained his weight at an ideal level for his size, a real challenge for most transplant recipients because prednisone increases appetite and makes it all too easy to gain weight without trying. And, as evidenced by his blood cholesterol, he kept a fairly tight rein on the fatty foods and dairy products.

Acknowledging how difficult it is for so many of us to eat properly and maintain normal weight, we encourage recipients to work with the registered dieticians who assist our transplant team. We try to keep the restrictions as relaxed as possible, but we are acutely aware that diet makes an enormous difference in the overall recovery and rehabilitation after heart transplantation. If one does not follow a prudent diet, it is, unfortunately, easy to gain twenty or thirty pounds during the first two years following surgery. Sensible dietary modification also includes restricting sodium intake, for not only does prednisone promote weight gain, it also increases salt and fluid retention, which, in turn, elevate blood pressure. Since cyclosporine further raises blood pressure, restricting dietary sodium—in the form of salt added to food during cooking or at the table—is absolutely required. Excess caloric intake, added to the potential effects of the antirejection medications, also may lead to developing diabetes. Thus, for many reasons, our dietary goal is to maintain near ideal body weight, along with limiting the daily intake of saturated fats, concentrated sweets, and salt. Fortunately, these are health-promoting dietary principles for everyone, regardless of whether they have had a heart transplant.

Approximately 75 percent of heart recipients are able to return to their previous occupation or activities, and our experience is that most do so. It is not usually necessary to impose any specific restrictions regarding life-style that would not also be good health practices for the average person. Probably, what is most different for heart transplant recipients is their daily requirement for maintenance medications. They must comply rigidly with the schedule required for taking these powerful drugs and be on the lookout for potential complications that may arise. Well-informed recipients are best able to help us identify early, and treat effectively, complications such as organ rejection, infection, or adverse drug side-effects. All of this said, one of the truly remarkable and satisfying results of modern advances in heart transplantation is that most recipients are capable of living a full, fairly unencumbered life after their surgery.

Coping with Complications

Approximately four and a half months after his transplant, Rob started feeling a little punk—an expression we use when a recipient isn't feeling quite right. He first felt it while jogging—the gradual onset of mild shortness of breath. Although otherwise he felt perfectly well, a routine heart biopsy showed moderate transplant rejection. An echocardiogram the same day showed that his overall heart function was still normal despite the rejection. "This is very often the case with mild to moderate rejection," we told Rob. "We'd like to give you three days of intravenous steroids. We can do it as an outpatient. You'll just come to the hospital for a short visit each day, and still go to school. I hope you'll be able to carry on pretty much as normal."

Ten days later we repeated the biopsy and found that the rejection episode had resolved. Rob's symptoms had also vanished. Since that time, he has been free of rejection. This is also fairly typical, but we still keep our fingers crossed for good luck. The period of greatest risk for rejection is the first three to six months, but it never fully goes away. With each month that passes, however, we are more confident that the immune barrier has been successfully bridged.

After transplantation, most recipients have periods when there are complications: organ rejection, infection, other medical problems. During these times, it is normal to feel frightened, depressed, or uncertain. Fortunately, the episodes usually resolve favorably, as they did for Rob Richmond. Treatment is available for the medical problems, while support and counseling are there to help patients cope with the emotional distress.

SIDE-EFFECTS OF CYCLOSPORINE

The side-effects of immunosuppressives are explained in greater detail in Chapter 3. For heart recipients, two especially troublesome side-effects of long-term cyclosporine therapy are hypertension (high blood pressure) and abnormalities of kidney function. More than 80 percent of heart recipients taking cyclosporine develop hypertension, as compared to less than 50 percent of kidney or liver recipients. As yet, we do not know why this difference exists. Most new recipients have some rise in blood pressure within the first ninety days following surgery. At times, two or three different medications may be required to control the hypertension. Approximately half of all recipients also have some abnormality of kidney function after the first year of taking cyclosporine. Fortunately, the problem usually does not worsen progressively and often improves as we are able to decrease the cyclosporine dosage. If an abnormality of kidney function is noted on blood or urine tests we immediately begin to adjust medication dosage, and follow up with frequent laboratory tests to make certain the problem is kept under control.

INFECTION

Organ rejection wasn't the only complication Rob had to overcome. About eighteen months after the transplant, he began feeling nauseated and tired. He had difficulty eating and lost ten pounds. His mother noticed that his eyes were slightly yellow. She worried that he might have hepatitis and took him to the transplant clinic. As soon as we saw him, we also were concerned and ordered blood tests, which came back positive. But was the liver inflammation due to an infection or to the medications? Adjustments were made in his drugs. Over a month went by and he still had evidence of hepatitis, so we brought him into the hospital for a liver biopsy. It came back showing that he had a very mild case of hepatitis. We kept his medication regimen the same, and Rob

went home to recover. In a few months, the hepatitis resolved, and his spirits improved.

Because of the daily immunosuppressive medications, we
are always concerned about potential infectious complications
(see Chapter 4). But the first six months after surgery are most
critical, because the body is still recovering and the immunosuppressive doses are still rather high. Even though the majority of infections are caused by viruses, which resolve on
their own without treatment, we are always concerned about
bacterial infections, which require antibiotic treatment. It is,
therefore, essential that any sign of infection—whether it is a
fever, or just feeling a little punk—be reported promptly to the
transplant team. The earlier we investigate these episodes, the
easier it is to develop strategies for handling them. Overall,
regardless of the offending source, *preventing* a serious infection is far preferable to trying to manage it once it develops.
Please review carefully the suggestions in Chapter 4; we rely
on the recipient and family to alert us to the *earliest* signals of
trouble. Once alerted, we can undertake appropriate diagnostic
studies and institute treatment if needed. We also routinely
prescribe certain oral antimicrobial medications, like Bactrim
and Nystatin (an antifungal drug), as preventive measures.

The Long Term

The majority of transplant recipients—now over 75 percent—
can expect to live five or more healthy, active years with their
new heart. In medical terms, we consider five-year survival to
be a benchmark point for long-term survival, although we are
acutely aware that for a relatively young person this is still not
a normal life span. Fortunately, the art and science of heart
transplantation are advancing steadily and rapidly. Considering that Christiaan Barnard's first operation was performed
just over two decades ago, to us the advances in our field seem
remarkable. Nevertheless, despite improvements in surgical
technique, immunosuppression, and the prevention and management of infection, each year a small percentage of recipients

die. At most transplant centers, acute rejection continues to be the most common cause of death during the first one to two years following surgery. The second most common cause is infection, which accounts for between 20 and 40 percent of deaths. Although the risk of acquiring a fatal infection has decreased enormously since we began using cyclosporine, all recipients remain at some risk because their normal defenses are reduced.

The third important cause of mortality is chronic rejection which fails to abate despite our varied options for immuno-suppression. This process may produce chronic damage to the heart muscle and result in slow, progressive deterioration of overall heart function. Increasingly, we are also seeing the progressive narrowing of the coronary arteries that supply blood to the transplanted heart. This process is felt to be a manifestation of chronic, low-grade rejection; the arterial narrowing is usually progressive and diffuse, and cannot be treated with bypass surgery or angioplasty (a new, less invasive method for clearing blocked arteries). It may appear as early as the first year, or it may take many years to develop. Chronic rejection involving the heart muscle or the coronary arteries accounts for between 10 and 20 percent of all deaths after heart transplantation, but almost always occurs after the first three to five years.

Fairly uncommonly—probably among no more than 5 percent of recipients—other problems may arise, including cancers. The exact relationship of these illnesses to the transplant is not fully understood, but they are presumed to be related to long-term immunosuppression. There are also deaths due to accidents, and a small number of "miscellaneous causes," often entirely unrelated to the transplant.

Future Directions

Despite the formidable advances that have been made over the last two decades, a number of significant obstacles remain to even more widespread application of heart transplantation.

First, we must find better ways to suppress the immune system. At this moment the focus is on finding immunosuppressive drugs capable of preventing rejection without increasing the risk of infection. Although cyclosporine has had a tremendous impact on survival by allowing more precise immunosuppression than was available with azathioprine and prednisone alone, it is neither entirely effective in preventing rejection nor without major side-effects. Currently, an enormously active and promising area is the search for better immunosuppressive agents.

Second, we need to develop a suitable mechanical heart that can act as the bridge between dying from heart disease and finding a suitable donor organ. *The major short- and long-term problem in the field of heart transplantation remains the lack of suitable donor organs.* In most transplant programs, approximately 20 percent of the patients waiting for a new heart die before a suitable donor heart becomes available. The number of people who could benefit from heart replacement, but who do not receive a transplant, is actually even larger, since many patients are not ever listed because of the acute shortage of donors. Moreover, the donor shortage can only be expected to worsen in the upcoming decade, as more centers become capable of performing heart transplantation while end-stage heart disease continues as a major killer. Although over the last decade public awareness regarding the donation of organs has increased, and "required request laws" have been enacted in many states, in the foreseeable future the number of available donor hearts will always fall far short of the need.

Two approaches currently are being pursued to help alleviate the organ shortage. The first is the use of nonhuman donors. Efforts are currently under way to evaluate the potential for transplanting hearts from other species such as pigs, sheep, or chimpanzees. Unfortunately, to date, the problem of rejection with nonhuman organs has been insurmountable. Perhaps improved immunosuppressive agents might someday be capable of overcoming this barrier. If this approach comes to fruition, we will have to tackle the ethical and moral implications of raising other species for the purpose of harvesting their organs to preserve human life.

At this moment it appears that the more likely long-term solution is developing a viable artificial heart. So far, the artificial heart, like the Jarvik-7 that made headlines in Salt Lake City, has been tried in only a very small number of patients, and only for several months, in experimental settings. Generally, the results have not been acceptable for more widespread use, so the approach is confined to being a temporary bridge to transplantation for people who are critically ill. The feasibility of a long-term or permanent artificial heart continues to be debated. At present, the need for large, external tubes to supply power, along with the power console itself, prevents the recipient from leading any sort of normal life. Work is meanwhile under way to develop a totally implantable device with its own battery-powered vest, which would enhance potential long-term usefulness. While developmental designs have improved dramatically over the last five years, a satisfactory totally implantable heart that would permit an individual to resume a nearly normal life is probably many years in the future. Unless we can overcome the rejection of nonhuman hearts, a mechanical device ultimately is the only approach that could supply enough hearts for the many thousands of persons who die each year from end-stage heart disease.

> We cannot accurately predict how long Rob Richmond will live with his new heart. Five years? Based on the results since cyclosporine, that seems very likely. Will he marry and have children of his own? Only time will tell, of course, but that is our hope for him.

Heart-Lung Transplantation

There are many people with long-standing heart failure who cannot benefit from heart transplantation alone, because their lungs are damaged as a result of their heart disease. In addition, there are others suffering from severe lung diseases, such as pulmonary fibrosis or cystic fibrosis, that cause progressive pulmonary scarring or recurrent infections. Over a period of many years, these illnesses may produce heart failure, too. Until recently, burdened by failure of both heart and lungs, these people had no hope for long-term survival.

For more than thirty years, there has been considerable interest in the concept of replacing lungs and heart together in one combined transplant procedure. Because of the enormous technical difficulties involved, the idea remained dormant until the late 1960s and early 1970s, when a few highly experimental heart-lung transplants were attempted. Unfortunately, our ability to prevent organ rejection was still not up to the task, and no one lived more than a week. Through the 1970s, research and animal experimentation produced improvements in both surgical and immunosuppressive techniques, so that, in March 1981, the first successful heart-lung transplant was performed at Stanford Medical Center—a milestone, providing new life for a forty-five-year-old woman, that opened the door for others with severe, combined heart and lung disease. Three factors make heart-lung replacement perhaps our greatest challenge in the field of organ transplantation. The first is the technical problems in performing the surgery. Second, it is difficult to diagnose rejection early, when it can be best treated. Third, there is a *very* short supply of suitable heart-lung donors, so that potential recipients sometimes wait a considerable period of time. Thus these recipients are often severely debilitated at the time of surgery.

Currently, there are several different lung conditions that produce severe heart failure that can be treated with heart and lung transplantation, along with conditions that can be treated with lung replacement, which we describe next. These conditions result in *pulmonary hypertension,* in which the walls of the lungs' tiny arteries thicken and narrow. This increases resistance to blood flowing from the right side of the heart into the lungs. Like any muscle forced to perform against resistance, the right side of the heart initially adjusts to its task by thickening (hypertrophy) and enlarging (dilation). Over time, however, the added burden causes the heart muscle to deteriorate, producing the same symptoms of heart failure experienced by Rob Richmond: weakness, fatigue, shortness of breath, fluid retention, and so on. If left untreated by heart-lung transplantation, in about five years death eventually comes, either from a sudden disturbance of heart rhythm or more gradually from overall organ failure.

Patients with advanced pulmonary hypertension due to one of a number of possible illnesses are ideally suited for heart-lung transplantation. Some are children born with a heart defect that ultimately would progress to fatal pulmonary hypertension if not treated with organ replacement. Although people with pulmonary hypertension make up the largest single group for heart-lung replacement, there also is a broad spectrum of lung diseases that cause progressive respiratory failure followed by heart failure. These include advanced emphysema, interstitial fibrosis (progressive scarring of the lung tissues due to unknown causes), and advanced cystic fibrosis. As we describe later in this chapter, some people affected by these conditions may be able to benefit from lung transplantation alone, provided their cardiac function has not deteriorated. However, if heart failure has developed, combined heart-lung transplantation is required, since lung replacement alone does not solve the problem of a failing, overworked heart.

Matching Recipient and Donor
Only 10 percent of all cardiac donors can provide lungs as well. Primarily, this is because accidents that cause brain death often damage the lungs, or because the lungs are damaged during prolonged support on a ventilator. Since donor organs are so scarce, it is not unusual for a potential recipient to wait more than two years for heart-lung transplantation. And since there are so few heart-lung replacements available, the criteria for selecting recipients are understandably very strict, substantially more so than those for heart transplantation alone. In general, heart-lung recipients must be under age forty-five,

and except for their heart and lung disease must be in excellent physical health. Prior kidney failure, diabetes, extensive prior chest surgery, or other complicating medical conditions eliminate a potential recipient from consideration. And, since the new lungs are susceptible to infection and injury, former smokers must demonstrate the ability to remain strictly off tobacco. Psychological factors are very important also, as recipients must participate actively in their postoperative rehabilitation and faithfully follow their medication schedules.

Proper matching of donor and recipient is critical in heart-lung transplantation. As with heart transplants, initial matching according to blood type and body size is performed. In addition, the new lungs must fit nearly perfectly inside the recipient's chest: lungs too large would be restricted in their movement, while lungs too small would leave space for fluid to pool and become infected. Using the chest X-ray, we carefully size the donor's lungs and the recipient's chest for the proper match.

As soon as a potential donor becomes available, we travel to the donor hospital to conduct a detailed evaluation. Obviously, we pay great attention to the donor's lung function: the chest X-ray must be clear of infection, the blood measurements of oxygen and carbon dioxide must be normal or very near normal. Microscopic and laboratory analysis of sputum (phlegm) also must show no evidence of infection. If the donor's heart and lungs pass all the tests, we call the recipient to the hospital and begin preparing for surgery.

Surgery

As for heart transplantation, both the harvesting and transplanting must be exquisitely coordinated, so that the recipient is in the operating room and ready to receive the replacement heart and lungs at the exact moment when the new organs arrive at the hospital. The transplant process follows much of what we described for cardiac replacement. First, the chest is opened, exposing the heart and major blood vessels, and the connections are made to the heart-lung machine, which will provide external support for oxygenating and circulating the blood. Now the new heart and lungs—transported and preserved on ice in a special salt solution—are ready to be installed in one replacement piece, the *heart-lung block*. Since the heart is connected to the lungs in several places, it is vital that the connections not be disturbed. Therefore, the blood vessels leading to and from the old heart are cut, disconnecting it from the body's vascular network. Next, the windpipe (trachea) is divided, permitting the diseased lungs to be removed with the diseased heart. Now, the remaining blood vessels are moved out of the way and the old heart and lungs lifted from the chest. For a brief, striking period, the chest is literally empty, except for the relatively few blood vessels connecting to the heart-lung machine.

The new heart and lung block is then brought into the operating room and removed from its transport container, and its blood vessels are thoroughly examined. Adjustments are made so that the donor's and recipient's blood vessels will match properly in size when sewn together. The heart and lung block is then lowered into the chest. Lying deepest within the chest cavity, the first connection made is to the windpipe; the edges of recipient and donor windpipes are sewn together securely, producing an airtight link. This is a particularly important and delicate part of the operation; the outer surface of the windpipe is covered with many small blood vessels which, if not properly attached, can bleed after surgery. Next, the blood vessels carrying "blue" unoxygenated blood from the body to the heart, and the aorta carrying "red" oxygenated blood from the heart to the body, are connected. Using the heart-lung machine, we can now begin rewarming, while also evacuating any air trapped in the heart and its blood vessels. As they fill with blood, the new heart and lungs turn pink with life. The rest of the operation proceeds like a heart transplant: medications are given to stimulate the heart and adjust its rate, and the anesthesiologist initiates breathing in the new lungs. In twenty to sixty minutes the new heart usually recovers and stabilizes, so that weaning from the heart-lung machine can slowly proceed. Medications are given to reverse the anticoagulant required for heart-lung bypass, and we spend considerable time checking for—and halting—any bleeding that may be occurring. Drainage tubes are inserted, the chest cavity is wired closed, and the skin is sutured together. Because the operation is so extensive, it leaves a considerable "raw surface" behind the heart. Bleeding after surgery can be a significant problem. During the first twenty-four hours after surgery, virtually all heart-lung recipients receive numerous transfusions, including blood platelets, which assist clotting. Nearly half will also require a second trip back to the operating room, to control postoperative bleeding, or to remove accumulated clotted blood.

Recovery

Following surgery, the new heart-lung recipient goes to the intensive care unit, where he or she will be isolated and protected from potentially infectious organisms. We must now be particularly protective of the recipient's transplanted respiratory system. Meticulous attention is paid to the details of caring for the windpipe and breathing tube. All new recipients require a mechanical respirator to control their breathing until they awake fully from the anesthesia, and some need the ventilator for an additional day or two. Weaning from the respirator usually is accomplished readily, as the recipient now has normal lungs.

Just as for heart transplant recipients, we begin immunosuppression immediately before surgery and continue indefinitely afterward. We try to minimize the dose of steroids, because these medications slow the healing process. In particular, it takes two to three weeks for healing of the connection between donor and recipient windpipes, during which time there is special concern about possible air leakage. We must also perform routine heart biopsies to check for possible heart rejection, and monitor closely the respiratory system for signs and symptoms of possible pneumonia or lung rejection.

Because the first signs may be very subtle, early detection

of lung rejection is a very special problem. It initially may manifest itself as a low-grade fever, slight difficulty in breathing, or a slight change on the daily chest X-rays. Analyzing the chest X-ray takes skill and experience, as the earliest warning may be a subtle, abnormal shadow that might signal either rejection or infection. Distinguishing between the two is absolutely critical, because their treatment takes us in opposite directions. In the face of rejection we temporarily increase the dose of immunosuppressive medications. If, however, the underlying cause of the X-ray shadow is infection, more immunosuppression is likely to aggravate the problem. Conversely, if lung rejection is improperly diagnosed as lung infection, treating by slightly decreasing the immunosuppression may make that worse. Thus, we must differentiate between infection and rejection in a very reliable manner.

Just as heart biopsies are used to detect heart rejection, we depend on lung biopsies to uncover lung rejection. Most lung biopsies can be obtained using a special instrument called the bronchoscope. After the patient is given a small amount of intravenous sedative (usually Valium), plus some local anesthetic sprayed into the throat, this flexible fiberoptic tool, about one-fourth of an inch in diameter, passes readily through the nose, down the windpipe, and into the lungs. With its telescopic capabilities we can both observe the transplanted lungs directly and obtain a small amount of tissue for laboratory analysis. The tissue, plus the direct visualization, provide an excellent way to differentiate infection from rejection. Rarely, the portion of the lung we wish to study is not accessible to the bronchoscope and, in these circumstances, we must make a small opening in the chest to perform an "open" lung biopsy. However, it is always our preference to use the bronchoscope to obtain a biopsy, since it can be performed without general anesthesia and with diminished risk of infection.

We treat lung rejection with steroid medications, usually methylprednisolone (Solu-Medrol), as with heart rejection. For reasons that still are not completely understood, heart-lung recipients experience far fewer and generally less severe episodes of heart rejection than do recipients of heart transplants alone. However, the heart and lungs do not necessarily have to experience rejection together, so it is possible for recipients to experience lung rejection without heart rejection or vice versa. Thus, the function of the heart and lungs must both be evaluated routinely. Over the long term, we are concerned about identifying and treating early the occasional person who slowly and insidiously develops lung rejection without apparent symptoms or abnormality on chest X-ray. If left untreated, the result can be destruction of the small air passages, a condition called *bronchiolitis obliterans,* in which there is slow and progressive obliteration of the lung passages leading to respiratory failure. With proper detection using serial pulmonary function studies, we can avoid this problem by increasing immunosuppression. Fortunately, bronchiolitis obliterans is not now a common problem among recipients.

The Horizon

Heart-lung transplantation is still a relatively new treatment for patients with advanced lung and heart disease. Because of its technical complexity, and because of the tremendous amount of postoperative care and attention that heart-lung recipients require, this type of transplantation is performed by only a small number of centers across the nation. Furthermore, since only a very small number of donors are suitable for providing both heart and lungs, the number of patients who benefit from this treatment is extremely limited. For the recipients, however, the results generally have been excellent, including rehabilitation back to a good quality of life.

Transplanting the Lungs

The idea of replacing the lungs was first proposed by surgeons at the turn of the twentieth century, and by the late 1940s researchers were performing this complex feat on animals in the laboratory. The first human single-lung transplant, performed in 1963, unfortunately, was not a long-term success.

Over the next twenty years, only thirty-eight more such transplants were attempted, with the results being equally unsatisfactory. We seemed to be unable to overcome both the enormous technical complexities of the surgery and the postoperative rejection.

But because of the pressing need to help patients who otherwise would die from pulmonary disease, surgeons continued to work in the laboratory on this most daunting of operations. Throughout the 1960s and 1970s progress was being made in the field of thoracic (chest) surgery generally, and the new knowledge was later applied to lung transplantation. Surgeons working at a number of different institutions around the world were developing artful new techniques for reattaching severed or injured airways. With advances in maintaining adequate blood supply to the vital pulmonary structures, plus improved immunosuppression, the stage was set for attempting lung transplants once again. The Toronto Lung Transplant Group, under the direction of Dr. Joel D. Cooper, led the way. In 1983, they performed the first successful single-lung transplant. Soon other centers followed, so that worldwide about two hundred single-lung transplants have now been performed, along with approximately fifty double-lung operations. The recipients have been from one to sixty-three years of age. The success rate has gone up, with mortality for single-lung operations dropping from 35 percent in 1987 to less than 10 percent in 1989. Long-term survival is improving, too, with 85 percent or more of recipients alive one year after surgery and 75 percent or more alive after two or three years. Because the procedure is so new, data for the longer term are not available. Obviously, we are hopeful that the long-term results will soon approach those of other organ transplants.

Quality of life for recipients continues to improve as well, and in thinking about this aspect we must be mindful that all of these patients would have died in about eighteen months if they had not had their transplant. After rehabilitation, most recipients are off oxygen, and can return to their normal activities. Generally, they experience no more than two episodes of infection during the first year after surgery, and rejection is typically well controlled. Also, there has been an extremely low occurrence of long-term impairment of lung function.

Double-lung replacement is required when leaving one abnormal lung—for instance, in individuals with cystic fibrosis—is likely to be a source of future, lethal infection. Here again the Toronto group broke ground, performing the first double-lung transplant in 1987. This operation is more difficult than single-lung surgery, so while an ever increasing number of patients are undergoing single-lung replacement, double-lung transplantation remains a more daunting and uncertain prospect. However, while the success of double-lung replacement has been somewhat less than that for single-lung operations, it still is quite encouraging.

Surgery and Recovery

There are three options for lung transplantation: single, double and, as already described, heart-lung. In the single-lung operation, one native lung and the heart remain; in double-lung surgery, only the heart remains; and in the heart-lung operation, both lungs and the heart are transplanted from a single donor. Single- and double-lung transplantation are also termed *isolated lung transplantation.* Normally, we have two lungs, but for most people one is sufficient for a normal life. Thus, if there is no infection in the remaining native lung, we often can replace only one organ and still have a successful transplant. The body seems to cooperate readily: after a single-lung transplant over 90 percent of the blood flow from the heart goes to the new, healthy organ. Similarly, the body adapts by preferentially aerating the new lung, rather than the old one. By about three months after surgery, the lung function of a single-lung-transplant recipient is much like that of someone who has had one lung removed.

The success of any of these operations depends on maintaining not only good lung function but also that of the heart, which must quickly adapt to the newly replaced lung(s). Along with overcoming rejection, preventing heart failure postoperatively has been an enormous obstacle. A third major difficulty is maintaining the replacement lung or lungs in good condition after they are cut off from the donor's circulation. Deprived of oxygen and nutrients from the donor's bloodstream, the lungs are extremely sensitive to injury. Once removed from the donor, the lungs quickly build up toxic waste products. With current methods for organ preservation, the lungs must be transplanted within six hours to ensure a successful operation. A fourth complicating factor is related to normal lung physiology. During the immediate period after surgery there is a tendency for fluid to build up. To prevent this complication, the patient's fluid intake must be restricted for the first five to seven days following transplantation.

In the process of removing the donor organ(s), the normal nerve supply is disturbed, resulting in a lung with reduced sensitivity to potential airborne irritants. The cough reflex is diminished, so the recipient must be actively stimulated, and reminded, to cough to eliminate unwanted water and inhaled particles. Additionally, disturbing the nerve supply reduces the normal ability to increase respiratory rate when the body needs more oxygen. Fortunately, this problem diminishes over the first three to six months after surgery. The way in which the body adapts over time is not fully understood, but it means that lung-transplant recipients are soon able to live a relatively normal life—working, dancing, even cross-country skiing.

Much of what we have already said about heart and heart-lung transplantation applies to lung replacement as well. Donors and recipients are matched for blood type and body size. The same drugs are used to prevent rejection, except that in the immediate postoperative period we avoid using steroids. This seems to help prevent complications related to healing of the attachments between the donor's and the recipient's airways. By about three weeks after surgery, however, recipients are usually receiving a standard three-drug regimen of cyclosporine, azathioprine, and prednisone. A number of laboratory techniques are available to assess rejection, including lung scan, biopsy, and a new laser test that measures blood flow in the lungs. Signs of rejection include shortness of breath and fever. Since a recipient is likely to live far from the transplant center, at home we monitor rejection with a relatively simple machine that measures lung function. This pulmonary function testing is performed on a regular basis, and a decline on two successive tests prompts return to the hospital for further testing.

The Future

Over the last decade, the possibility of transplanting the lungs has become a reality. For patients with both heart and lung failure, heart-lung transplantation is now available; for those with lung failure only, either single- or double-lung replacement is an option. And, while double-lung surgery is still considered experimental or investigative, the results are sufficiently encouraging to open a window of hope where there was none before. The hope is that further advances in preserving donor organs, preventing rejection, and improving surgical techniques will enhance the applicability of this life-saving therapy. Since a person can function well with a single lung, on the horizon, perhaps, is allowing living related donors—as in kidney transplantation—to provide an organ for a loved one. Another application may be to provide a life-saving opportunity when someone suffers a potentially fatal accidental injury to the chest. Thus, while lung transplantation is in its infancy, it holds great promise. And like an infant, it is undergoing a phase of rapid growth and development on its way to full-fledged maturity as a life-saving transplant procedure.

Kidney, Pancreas, and Liver Transplantation

Transplanting the Kidney

Ken Laughlin's kidney disease was an inherited time bomb waiting to go off. When Ken was twenty his father died from kidney failure. When Ken became ill, he was thirty-seven, with kids, a wife, and a job in the high tech industry.

Ken, it turned out, had inherited his father's problem, polycystic kidney disease. Ten years after the onset of his disease, now divorced with three teenage boys living at home, Ken was suffering from kidney failure. He first came to our hospital to participate in a study of a relatively new drug, EPO, that works to prevent the anemia caused by kidney failure. By that time he had been on dialysis for over a year, and not been feeling terribly well. He was tired all the time, had trouble sleeping, and wanted very much to be free of dialysis. "I feel tied down, caged in by the dialysis machine," he said. "I just can't seem to work full time and keep up with the boys." When we brought up the option of getting a new kidney, Ken was enthusiastic.

Today, the replacement of the human kidney is almost routine at major medical centers throughout the world. But only a few decades ago it was no more than a dream for people in the final stages of renal disease. At that time, dialysis also was in its infancy. Now, for Ken Laughlin and others like him, a successful transplant—with an almost normal quality of life afterward—is a reality. The success we anticipate for Ken is also a model toward which we strive when replacing other organs and tissues.

Renal disease is unique in that there are three different treatments available for patients with what is called end-stage disease. There are hemodialysis and peritoneal dialysis, in which waste products are filtered from the body; and there is organ replacement. Over the course of their illness, most people avail themselves of more than one of these options. Like Ken, most transplant recipients have a period of time on dialysis before, and sometimes after, their transplant. Age, medical problems, and most of all, personal considerations regarding work and quality of life, determine the appropriate choice of treatment option.

Dialysis

Dialysis was invented to cleanse the blood of waste products that build up when the kidneys do not function normally. The process involves passing a patient's blood through a machine equipped with compartments that are separated by a semi-permeable membrane. The membranes act as filters, permitting impurities to pass out of the bloodstream into a purifying solution (the dialysate fluid) in the chambers. During the dialysis session excess fluid is squeezed out by mechanical pressure that forces water out of the bloodstream. In this way unwanted water is removed with the waste products.

However, dialysis does not perform many of the kidneys' other vital functions, including stimulating the body to produce red blood cells. Consequently, people on dialysis develop anemia. Fortunately, a new drug, erythropoietin or EPO, is now available to take over the kidneys' role in stimulating red cell production. We are still learning about EPO—as we mentioned, Ken Laughlin came to the hospital to be part of an EPO study—but from what we already know, it appears to be helpful in ameliorating much of the anemia associated with renal failure. With EPO and future advances, we expect that people on dialysis will enjoy better appetite, increased energy and sex drive, and a better overall sense of well-being. Nonetheless, life on dialysis is restricting in many ways. It is very time-consuming, so it often interferes with work. There are rather strict dietary dos and don'ts—certain foods must be avoided altogether, and the intake of others carefully monitored. There are restrictions with regard to. travel, since three-to-four-hour dialysis sessions are required about three times a week. All of this means, as Ken said, feeling tied to the machine. And there are potential medical difficulties, especially the Achilles' heel of hemodialysis—establishing and maintaining access to the bloodstream. This is a special problem for people with diabetes or peripheral vascular disease, for the elderly, whose blood vessels are fragile, and for children, whose blood vessels are small. Moreover, despite continual improvements in the technology, each year about 10 percent of people on dialysis die, usually because of cardiovascular problems like heart attack and stroke.

The Transplant Option

It is fair to say that people on dialysis never feel totally normal. After a while it is common to want the freer life that can be enjoyed with a successful kidney transplant; a life where one feels well and is no longer restricted in terms of travel or diet. Nevertheless, as with all transplants, there are two principal obstacles to success: rejection and infection. As we have discussed previously, these problems are related. Fortunately, with improved immunosuppression we have learned highly effective ways of maintaining the replacement kidney while keeping up adequate immune defenses against contagious disease. For kidney recipients, especially, after the initial high doses of immunosuppression, years follow in which only rather modest, long-term maintenance drug therapy is required. During this time, the body tends to accept the new organ, and becomes used to the medications.

Immediately after kidney transplant surgery, the mainstays of drug therapy are prednisone and cyclosporine, and sometimes azathioprine. These drugs and their side-effects have been discussed already, but it is worthwhile to emphasize that cyclosporine has been enormously beneficial for two reasons: first, in improving long-term survival of the new kidney, and second, in permitting the rapid tapering off of the prednisone. Nowadays, at the end of one week, we are at the dose that people used to reach at six to eight months after surgery. This has meant avoiding many of the unwanted side-effects and complications of high doses of steroids—puffy face, weight gain, bone softening, high blood pressure, and cataracts. Nevertheless, it is critically important to remember that, as long as the transplanted organ is functioning, some level of maintenance immunosuppression is necessary. If at any point a recipient stops taking the medications rejection can occur—even ten or fifteen years after the transplant.

> While he was on peritoneal dialysis, Ken complained of the things that seem to bother everyone: dry skin, itching, dietary restrictions. Even on the EPO he was anemic. He also had problems with high blood pressure, and his hearing was declining. One good thing was that even after months on the dialysis machine, he had managed to avoid a single episode of peritonitis, an infection associated with that type of dialysis. It showed that he was very conscientious about following directions for his medical care, and for his hygiene generally.
>
> Ken very much wanted to get back to his normal work routine. He was sensitive about any interruption in his income, as he still expected to put his youngest son—age fourteen—through college. He thought a lot about that, and worried about the job he was doing as a single parent. Getting off dialysis seemed critical to the task of finishing raising his children. He also felt bad that his oldest boy was bearing so much of the family responsibility—going to college and working, being available to help

out around the house—because of his illness. It was time to find Ken a new kidney.

The Donor

There are two sources of kidneys for transplantation: living related donors and cadaveric donors. Living donors are usually members of the recipient's immediate family, like a parent, brother or sister, or child. Employing a living related donor permits scheduling the operation ahead of time. More important it improves the likelihood of a successful transplant, since genetically related individuals have a better chance of making a good tissue match. In fact, depending on the closeness of the match, between 85 and 95 percent of these transplants are functioning at the end of one year. In the best situation, where siblings share the same genetic material (where they are HLA identical; see Chapter 2), one-year survival of the new kidney approaches 95 percent.

Before a transplant from a living related donor can be performed, it is essential to be sure that the donor is healthy, without evidence of high blood pressure, diabetes, or abnormal renal function. The donor's medical evaluation includes a complete medical history, a thorough physical examination, and in addition to some basic laboratory tests (blood and urine analysis, EKG, chest X-ray), an intravenous pyelogram (IVP) to be sure the donor has two normally functioning kidneys.

By the time kidney donors enter the hospital, they already have gone through all these tests. We leave one last test for the day before surgery—an angiogram, which is an X-ray of the blood vessels supplying the kidneys. Under local anesthesia a long thin tube, called a catheter, is introduced into the artery in the groin, and a special dye is injected that permits the radiologist to examine the kidneys' circulation. Except for a rather unpleasant, but very brief, hot flush when the dye is injected, the procedure is fairly painless. The study is important because it provides a road map for the transplant surgeons. Since it is easier to remove the kidney with the fewest blood vessels, the choice of which side to operate on depends on the results of the angiogram.

After the angiogram, the remainder of the preoperative time in the hospital is spent preparing the donor and his or her kidneys for surgery. Large amounts of fluid are administered intravenously, the skin on the side of the operation is shaved and washed, food and water are withheld after midnight, and some preoperative sedatives are given. The next day, the donor and recipient operations usually are coordinated to take place at essentially the same time. After being put under general anesthesia, the donor is turned to expose the flank with the kidney that is to be removed. An incision is made over the tip of the twelfth or last rib, and a portion of the bone is removed. The donor kidney is carefully exposed, its blood vessels and ureter are identified, and when all is ready, it is separated from its blood supply and removed from the body. Now, it must be rapidly flushed with a cold solution to preserve it until it is reconnected to the recipient's blood supply. Not long after the kidney is delivered to the recipient's nearby operating suite, the donor's wound will be sewn together and he or she will be allowed to wake up.

Like any surgery, the donor's operation causes substantial postoperative discomfort. Actually, it is likely to be more uncomfortable than the recipient's procedure, so it is not unusual that by the next morning it is the recipient who walks down the hall to visit the donor. However, this pain after surgery can be controlled with medication, and in two or three days the donor is usually feeling better. It will also take several days for bowel function to return so food can be eaten. Most kidney donors leave the hospital on about the fifth day after their operation, sooner in almost every case than the recipient. The most common problem, which is relatively minor, is difficulty in passing urine immediately after surgery; this may require placing a catheter in the bladder for one or two days. Serious complications are extremely rare. Except for avoiding potential injury to the remaining kidney, the donor can expect to live normally.

Normal life does not resume immediately, however. Recovery takes some time, adding further inconvenience to the act of donation. The same general rules described for the recipient apply for the donor: bathe or shower without restriction, walk up to the limit of discomfort, avoid heavy lifting (like picking up small children, carrying large bundles), wait about two weeks before driving, expect that it will take about six weeks to get back to work. Even more than for the recipient, expect that the incision will cause a nagging ache—which can be quite discouraging—for several weeks. Plan to make relatively brief postoperative medical visits at about six weeks, one year, and then once a year to have kidney function evaluated. This evaluation can be performed at the transplant center, or by a community physician.

One kidney is enough for good health and a normal life. Insurance companies recognize this fact, so a person's life and health insurance rates do not change after donating a kidney. The most common long-term problems are a small increase in the risk of developing high blood pressure or excreting protein in the urine. Mostly, however, donors lead completely normal lives. Six or eight weeks after surgery their activities are no longer limited. This includes an unrestricted diet, and for women, the expectation of normal pregnancy and childbirth. Because it is important to avoid accidents that might damage the remaining kidney, we caution against sky diving or very vigorous contact sports.

The decision as to whether to donate a kidney is a very personal one, and should be made only after careful consideration and discussion with family members, physician, and the transplant team. No one should ever be pressured to donate an organ.

The Recipient

Ken and his wife divorced about four months after he started on dialysis. Correctly or not, he believed their marital problems were directly related to stresses brought on by his illness. In the year after they broke up, one of his sons was working and going to college at night, while the one next in line was working, finishing high school, and getting ready for college. While their mom saw the boys regularly, Ken felt that most of the parenting burdens were on him—deciding on curfew, paying the bills, attending school events. He was concerned, too, that his children might someday develop the disease he had inherited from his father. So, for many reasons, all three boys participated in the pretransplant meetings and teaching sessions. The more we talked about it, the more everyone in the family became convinced. The eldest son offered to donate a kidney, but Ken declined.

The potential recipient of a renal transplant must have established, irreversible kidney disease, without evidence of active infection or cancer. Since noncompliance with the medical regimen is a major cause of long-term failure, a pretransplant psychiatric evaluation is important for determining whether the patient has the requisite motivation (see Chapter 5). We also look for ongoing alcohol or drug abuse, as these behaviors are known to have a negative impact on the future success of the operation. If a patient has a prior history of substance abuse, we generally require a one-year period of sobriety before considering transplantation. With major advances in the success of kidney transplantation, the age factor is diminishing in importance. While most recipients are between fifteen and fifty years old, transplants are now being provided for children under two, and in appropriate circumstances, for adults over sixty-five. In all respects Ken Laughlin was an ideal candidate.

The final step is a pretransplant family conference to review medical information and answer questions. At our hospital these meetings include a nephrologist (kidney specialist), a transplant surgeon, a psychiatrist, a primary nurse, a social worker, and a tissue typer. At this time, the recipient and family get a tour of the transplant unit and view a teaching video about transplantation. Now that everything is set, if we have a living related donor we schedule a date for surgery. Otherwise, the candidate is put on the waiting list for a kidney from a cadaveric donor. During the waiting period, the potential recipient keeps in regular contact with the transplant unit, supplying us with telephone numbers and a way to get in touch at any time of the day or night. When a donor became available for Ken, he was immediately called at home. When there was no answer, we remembered that he would probably be at his monthly visit to the nephrologist in the community. He was reached at the physician's office and in almost no time was on his way to the hospital. As we described in Chapter 1, we can even find someone at a rock concert!

While a living related transplant can be scheduled at the mutual convenience of donor and recipient, the waiting time for a cadaveric kidney varies. For someone with blood type A the waiting period is approximately six months; for blood type B it is six to twelve months; and for blood type 0 the waiting period is often more than one year. During the waiting period, the potential recipient's status is reviewed weekly, so that each time a kidney becomes available he or she is considered for a match. While waiting for an organ, the patient must "stay in training." This means refraining from smoking, maintaining normal body weight, and keeping to an appropriate exercise program.

The Operation

Because he was an unsensitized blood type A, Ken wasn't on the waiting list very long—he was first listed at the end of March and had his operation on April 26. We reached him about 3 P.M.; he went home to get some things and at approximately 6 P.M. was driven to the hospital by his middle son. There was no operating room time available that night, because another transplant was being performed, so his transplant was scheduled for the next day. Nevertheless, he got a good night's sleep, and the next morning a huge right polycystic kidney was taken out, and a new, healthy kidney was put in.

Transplanting the kidney requires general anesthesia, which begins in most operating rooms with the injection of a rapidly acting barbiturate into the bloodstream through an intravenous line. Within seconds the prospective recipient goes from talking with his or her doctor to being fast asleep. The patient's next impression is of gradually emerging from sleep when the operation is over. Typically, the surgery takes about four hours—time that is all unknown to the recipient, but that can be long indeed for family and friends.

The new kidney is not placed in the same location as the native kidneys, primarily because it is hard to surgically attach the replacement kidney to the existing blood vessels—which are high in the abdomen and quite far back. Instead, surgeons have learned to place the transplanted kidney low in the abdomen, in the hollow of the pelvic bone, and to connect it to the blood vessels that pass downward toward the legs. After surgery one can sometimes feel the new kidney deep beneath the skin in the lower abdomen, whereas it is unusual to be able to feel our native kidneys. A transplanted kidney is thus somewhat more exposed than normal, so it is unwise for recipients to risk violent blows to the lower abdomen in such activities as tackle football or motorcycle riding.

In the operation, three anatomic structures are connected: an artery bringing blood to the kidney, a vein to let blood flow away from it, and a ureter to transport urine to the bladder. There are several technical variations in the way these structures can be connected, each one about equally efficient, so the choice depends on the preference of the transplant team and the particular circumstances of the recipient. In addition, as for Ken Laughlin, it may be important to remove the old kidney(s). This is done if they are infected or likely to pose future problems such as hypertension. Whenever possible we like to leave a native kidney, because it is capable of producing either a small amount of urine or other important substances, such as erythropoietin. This residual function also may be helpful if the transplant fails and the recipient returns to dialysis. Our preference generally is to remove one of the native kidneys, and use its native ureter for the attachment to the new kidney. At other centers, both native kidneys may be left in place, so that the ureter from the new kidney is attached directly to the bladder. Again, there is no single best way to perform the operation, so the choice of technique depends on the needs of the individual recipient and the approach that is most comfortable for the transplant team.

After the induction of anesthesia, a flexible tube called a Foley catheter is placed in the bladder to monitor the output of urine. The actual surgery now begins with a diagonal incision low on the abdominal wall, extending out to the flank. For technical reasons, it is somewhat easier to place the donor's right kidney on the recipient's left side, and vice versa. Therefore, the choice of the side on which we operate usually depends on the available donor kidney. Through this incision the native kidney is removed and the blood vessels supplying the leg are exposed. Meanwhile, the donor kidney, maintained on ice in the preserving solution, is brought to the operating room, where it is prepared for transplantation. When all is ready, it is removed from the cold and its blood vessels are rapidly sewn to those of the recipient. As soon as the clamps holding back blood flow are removed, the gray lifeless donor kidney swells and turns pink. Almost immediately it may begin making urine, filtering the bloodstream of toxic waste products and removing excess water. It is always a dramatic moment in the operating room when the lifeless organ revives.

After attaching the blood vessels, the surgeons then reconnect the ureter, either to the recipient's own drainage tube (a technique called a pyeloureterostomy) or directly to the bladder (a technique termed a neocystostomy). The fundamentals of the operation are now finished. Usually a rubber tube is left near the kidney and brought out through the skin, to drain the small amount of blood and serum that normally accumulates after any surgery. After careful inspection of the incision to make certain there is no bleeding, the wound is closed with sutures. We bury these stitches beneath the skin, so that only paper strips are visible on the skin surface. Then the anesthesia is gradually withdrawn, waking slowly begins, and it is time to move the patient to the recovery suite in the transplant unit. While there are risks to any major surgery, it is fair to say that this operation has become almost routine, with mortality from surgery now extremely rare. Recipients need not approach the operating room with fear that they will not survive the operation.

Recovery

Waking from anesthesia is like emerging from a dense fog. First, there are distant voices, along with some confusing visual images and a remote, but definite, sensation of pain. Gradually, the mind and the senses clear, and one becomes aware that the surgery is over. Still, much of the first night will be spent drifting in and out of sleep, as the pain medicines cause periods of greater and less sedation. Operations do cause pain. For someone who has not experienced this discomfort, it may be surprising how much it hurts. Another of the major advances of modern medicine has been to develop effective techniques for managing postoperative pain, especially during the first twenty-four to forty-eight hours when the discomfort is greatest.

> Ken seemed to feel better almost immediately after surgery. "I can't believe how good I feel," he said. "You told me I would feel wonderful, but it's even better than that." In part that good feeling was due to the high doses of steroids. By the second day after the operation he was virtually off pain medications. His incision healed quickly, his appetite improved, the itching went away. When the Foley catheter came out he had some difficulty urinating, so we gave him bethanechol chloride (Urecholine), a drug that stimulates the bladder to empty, which seemed to help. With his spirits high, Ken was up and about in the hallways, and planning on getting back home.

At first, it is not unusual for the new kidney to produce huge quantities of urine—in part because it has not yet regained the ability to limit that flow, and because even if a patient has been on dialysis there is a backlog of waste products to filter from the body. Sometimes, however, a new kidney may produce only small quantities of urine, a shock effect of being deprived of its normal blood supply. This condition, called acute tubular necrosis or ATN, occurs in about 20 percent of kidney transplants. It may last days, even occasionally weeks, and is understandably discouraging. It is helpful to be aware that essentially *all* kidney transplants recover from ATN, so that the absence of early function does not portend a serious problem. ATN causes some inconvenience, since a recipient may need to undergo dialysis or special tests—such as renal scans or even biopsies—to monitor the new kidney's function. It also may delay discharge from the hospital.

Whether the new kidney is functioning or not, there are certain routine events in the early postoperative course. If a pyeloureterostomy was performed, the Foley catheter can be removed on the day after surgery, whereas if the ureter was connected to the urinary bladder, the catheter will need to stay in place for about five days. By about the second day, the intravenous line will be disconnected. After any surgery there is a period when the digestive system does not handle food well, a condition called an *ileus*. With the return of normal intestinal motion, over the next few days it is possible to move gradually from clear liquids to solid food. Generally, kidney recipients are up, and walking the halls, by the morning after surgery. This activity gets blood flowing in the legs and the lungs breathing deeply. Following surgery, to keep secretions from pooling in the lungs, which might cause pneumonia, recipients are given instructions and assistance in deep breathing exercises and coughing. Also, on the morning after surgery the bandages usually can be taken off. With our operative technique there are no stitches waiting to be removed, only paper tapes across the incision. As the wound heals, these too will gradually come off, or fall off on their own. As mentioned earlier, there will be a tube, called a surgical drain, coming out through the skin near the incision. This tube clears fluid (called serum) from the deeper portions of the wound. When the drainage stops the drain is removed, in a brief and slightly uncomfortable procedure performed at the bedside. Gradually kidney function improves, so that the laboratory measures now familiar to people with renal disease—such as BUN and creatinine—start returning toward normal. There may be a few minor problems, like Ken Laughlin's difficulty in urinating when the Foley catheter came out, which can be treated readily. Only very rarely are there more serious postoperative complications; these are understandably frustrating and frightening, but they can almost always be corrected.

More often than not, the first week after kidney transplantation is a grace period when things keep getting better. However, the clear sailing can be misleading, since the majority of kidney recipients have times in the hospital, or soon after discharge, when the functioning of their new kidney diminishes. These episodes are almost always successfully treated by adjusting the medication regimen. By far the two most common causes of diminished renal function are rejection and the toxic side-effects of cyclosporine. About 70 percent of recipients will manifest some signs of organ rejection, and most will also have some evidence of cyclosporine toxicity. Both problems manifest themselves as decreasing urinary output and rising laboratory values of blood BUN and creatinine. Usually we treat both problems simultaneously, by adding extra doses of steroids.

Relatively infrequently, there are other underlying causes for diminishing renal function, which can be diagnosed by routine blood and other studies. If, after the patient receives more steroids, renal function continues to deteriorate, it becomes essential to determine the underlying cause—especially if the choice is between rejection and cyclosporine toxicity. In the first instance, one needs more immunosuppression, in the second, less—a difference that is obviously of considerable importance. The next test to help distinguish between these possibilities is a kidney biopsy, usually performed at the hospital bedside under local anesthesia. While the procedure causes mild discomfort, it is more frightening than painful, and because of its new location it is less uncomfortable than the biopsy of a native kidney. Unfortunately, even this procedure may not always provide a definitive answer. Nevertheless, a transplant team is prepared for such ambiguous information and has strategies for dealing with the problem.

The important message is that most recipients can expect to have some problems getting adjusted to their new organ, and that after the initial discharge it may be necessary to return to the hospital for one or more additional short stays. New drugs may be needed, and the doses of the antirejection medications will probably require adjustment. This fine-tuning is a *normal* part of recovering. Again, the point to remember is that the vast majority of renal transplants are successful. Thus, the statement that someone is suffering rejection, while understandably sounding disturbing, is not cause for undue alarm. Almost every case of rejection can be reversed, and the other causes of abnormal renal function also can be corrected. Well over 90 percent of recipients leave the hospital with a kidney functioning sufficiently to keep them off of dialysis.

> Because of his reaction to the cyclosporine, Ken's creatinine came down a little more slowly than we hoped. We had started him on 500 milligrams twice a day, but had to reduce the dose to 350 milligrams twice a day before he could leave the hospital. To compensate for this change, we added azathioprine. He also had some difficulty with high blood pressure, which required adding another medication. Generally a fairly laid back person, Ken seemed to take these changes in stride. Mostly, he felt in a hurry to get home to his boys.

Kidney transplant recipients generally stay in the hospital between ten and fourteen days after surgery, and a few stay longer when their postoperative course is more complicated.

As discharge approaches there is much to learn about one's new life-style. The nurses on the transplant unit go over each of the medications, checking to be certain the recipient understands the doses and schedule for administration. We give each recipient a "Med Card" describing the medication regimen, which should be carried at all times and brought to medical appointments. As we have said before, *taking the medications according to prescription is absolutely essential for a successful transplant.* For about six weeks, recipients should also avoid heavy lifting or other activities that might place a significant strain on the surgical area. At home, you can bathe or shower, and peel off any remaining paper tape from the surgical area. As the discomfort eases, go for walks, climb stairs, engage in sexual relations, and generally do whatever feels comfortable. We advise waiting about two weeks before driving a car. The transplant team is available around the clock by telephone to deal with problems or to answer questions, and at discharge a follow-up appointment will be scheduled.

If the replacement organ did not come from a family member, every transplant recipient ponders questions about who the donor was, what he or she was like. While these questions are natural, transplant teams have learned, after much experience, that it is best not to satisfy this curiosity. The donor's family has a right to privacy, and the recipient enjoys the same protection. The donor's family is told only that the organ or organs were transplanted successfully, not the name or location of a particular recipient. Despite the scientific and medical advances that have made organ transplantation possible, there remains an element of mystery surrounding the human aspect, and we believe that some questions cannot, or should not, be answered.

Going Home

When Ken went home he was on three medications. At first his sons didn't want him to leave the house. It seemed they were worrying about everything. Ken enjoyed their attention—not usual from teenagers. For the first week, there were many visitors who brought food, helped clean up, and offered to do the shopping. But Ken wanted to be up and about. He took walks around the neighborhood, rode in the car to the store, and enjoyed not having to be on dialysis. In the clinic he soon was asking when he could go back to work. Based on our experience, the answer was in about two months. "Why not enjoy the vacation?" we asked. He smiled, and went back to being the more relaxed Ken we were accustomed to.

Even after discharge from the hospital, the work of maintaining a healthy kidney transplant goes on. Especially during the first three to six months, there probably will be regular changes in the medication regimen. The possibility of rejection continues, so recipients must come to the clinic for regular outpatient visits. Initially, this will be two or three visits each week, followed by a rapidly diminishing frequency. In addition to clinic visits, it may be important to have blood tests; for patients living far from their transplant center, these can be performed in the community. The results of the tests will be telephoned to the transplant unit. We think it is useful for recipients to be aware of their test results and to call the transplant unit *immediately* if they experience worrying physical symptoms. During the first few months after surgery, the special concerns and necessary medication adjustments are usually best handled by the transplant team, so that during this time most follow-up visits are to the transplant unit. Over time, this care can be provided by a community nephrologist, usually the doctor who treated the recipient before the transplant. It would be unfortunate and unnecessary to disturb this relationship, so after the first few months we encourage alternating visits between our transplant team and the community specialist.

For as long as someone has a kidney transplant, she or he faces certain special considerations regarding medical care that do not apply to the average person. The most important of these is the extraordinary importance of taking medications properly. Studies have shown that as time passes, it is unfortunately rather common to become lax about the drug regimen, often missing or capriciously adjusting the doses. As we have emphasized previously, the evidence is overwhelming that this behavior may lead to the loss of the replacement organ. Tragically, it happens that a recipient with an organ that has functioned well for many years begins to doubt the importance of the immunosuppression, stops taking the medications according to prescription, and then loses the organ to rejection. It appears that the most common cause of failed transplants in the late period is lack of compliance—sadly, a most preventable problem.

A second important consideration is weight gain, a problem for many people that is exacerbated by the medications. Not only does gaining unwanted pounds cause emotional stress, since we live in a society that sees thin as attractive, but it can also create serious health risks. For instance, the skeleton may already be weakened by disease, and obesity will further increase the risk of joint degeneration or fracture. Despite the many unproven claims in the tabloids, we all know there is no magic solution to weight control. Strict diets are essential. It is rare to see a transplant recipient successfully lose weight unless she or he is involved in a regular exercise program. On the positive side, most everyone who participates in regular exercise says that it improves their overall sense of well-being, providing a positive sense of self, with more energy for work, recreation, and personal relationships.

In Chapters 3 and 4, we discuss organ rejection and infection. In addition, for kidney transplant recipients, here are some specific signs to look for:

- Diminishing urine output in the face of normal fluid intake.
- Retention of fluid, especially noted as swelling of the feet or legs.
- Shortness of breath.

- Rising blood pressure.
- The return of any symptom experienced before the transplant.
- Fever, cough, or other sign of infection.

Should any of these symptoms arise, patients are instructed to call the transplant team or their community doctor.

As we have said, most kidney recipients enjoy a normal life-style after their transplant. Once the new kidney and the recipient are adjusted to each other, the goal of medical care soon becomes the same as for any other healthy person: preventing disease, along with detecting and successfully treating *early* problems that arise. For instance, women should have routine gynecologic evaluations and periodic mammograms. Both men and women should look for, and report promptly to their medical caregiver, any new skin lesion. In future years, the occasional visit to the transplant unit reminds recipients of these routine health maintenance chores. The community medical provider is available, as well, for this purpose. And, as mentioned previously, it is important to undertake a regular routine of exercise and physical fitness. Because most of us live busy lives, this is often best accomplished by a scheduled program at a health club. With the low doses of prednisone now routinely used for kidney transplantation, a recipient who works hard on physical fitness no longer need reveal himself or herself by a puffy face. It may take a bit more work than is required for others, but a kidney recipient now can look as healthy and as fit as anyone.

What If the Transplant Fails?

One of the important concerns of every recipient of a new kidney is what will happen if the transplant fails. For some this becomes almost an obsession, with every little event seen as a sign of kidney failure. A renal transplant may fail, of course, but rarely without warning, and generally over some time. If the concern begins immediately after the operation, the patient should keep in mind that it is extremely unusual for a replacement kidney never to regain function. So early problems, while inconvenient, should not be viewed with a sense of doom. As we mentioned, early rejection episodes are common and can almost always be treated successfully. Kidney transplants that are lost to rejection during the first three months tend to be lost to the second, third, or fourth episodes of rejection. After six months, acute rejection is quite unusual, unless medications are missed or their doses changed. If rejection occurs at this point, it is almost always chronic rejection (see Chapter 2), with urine output gradually diminishing and laboratory values of creatinine slowly rising. Chronic rejection may last months, or even years, before it finally destroys a kidney. Unfortunately, treatment for chronic rejection is not as successful as for acute rejection.

In addition to chronic rejection, slow deterioration of a transplanted kidney may be due to other causes, such as the narrowing of the blood vessels (called *renal artery stenosis*), which is usually associated with marked hypertension. In addition, some people develop a recurrence of their original illness; this is more common for some types of kidney disease than others. Furthermore, new kidney diseases can occur in the transplant. Because these various problems are treated differently, each recipient is evaluated individually—with laboratory tests, angiograms, biopsies. Managing declining renal function is much like treating the original kidney failure. At some point it usually is also necessary to establish access for hemodialysis or peritoneal dialysis. Most individuals who lose a kidney transplant are even more in a hurry to get a new one than people who have never been through the experience. Although care is taken to determine why the first kidney was lost, and to consider whether the loss is likely to occur again (making it unwise to go through an operation), most people are candidates for another replacement organ. Indeed, some people have returned for a third, fourth, or even, in extraordinary circumstances, a fifth transplant.

The speed with which people seek a second transplant is a testament to the quality of life they experienced while their first replacement kidney was working. Although dialysis permits people to survive and function adequately in daily activities—people who otherwise would die of renal disease—it brings an unfortunate dimunition of the quality of life. On the other hand, a successful kidney transplant provides an overall sense of well-being, with high energy and the freedom to live an essentially normal life.

Transplanting the Pancreas

It is estimated that each year 100,000 people learn they have diabetes requiring insulin replacement. Although the discovery of insulin in 1921 provided a means of controlling the elevated blood sugars that lead to acute attacks (termed *ketoacidosis*) that until then had been fatal, this only changed the long-term course of the disease. Today, as people with diabetes are living longer they are also increasingly suffering its long-term complications: kidney failure, blindness, diminished circulation, and loss of sensation in the extremities that may lead to amputation, heart attack, and stroke. After fifteen to twenty years, about half the people with insulin-dependent diabetes can expect to have one or more of these serious complications, reducing their life expectancy by about one-third, and making diabetes the third leading cause of death in the United States. While recent advances in the administration of insulin, such as the surgically implanted pump, are improving overall prognosis, it is rare to achieve constantly normal blood glucose (blood sugar) levels. Moreover, a number of problems, such as the daily burden of monitoring blood sugar, infections, and hypoglycemia (low blood sugar), still plague patients treated by the new techniques. Not surprisingly, only the most motivated and compliant people (perhaps about 10 percent) are able to follow the very strict regimens for controlling blood glucose. So, although recent evidence suggests that these new methods of strictly controlling blood sugar may arrest—even reverse—the progression of the diabetic complications, insulin-dependent diabetes remains a formidable problem. One hope is the new and rapidly progressing field of pancreas transplantation, which holds promise for providing a fully self-regulating source of insulin to effectively cure insulin-dependent diabetes.

> At age eleven, Janice suddenly found herself gaining weight and feeling thirsty all the time. Her parents took her to their family physician, and it was not long before the diagnosis of juvenile diabetes was confirmed. From that day onward, Janice lived with twice-daily insulin shots and a strictly controlled diet. Like many insulin-controlled diabetics, she was able to continue her schooling, pursue an active career as a teacher, marry, and start raising a family. Certainly there were times when her diabetes got in the way, but she learned ways to cope and never seemed to complain. Her condition was just a part of her.
>
> Then, in her early thirties, she began suffering the degenerative kidney disease that is all too common after about twenty years of needing insulin. By the time she was thirty-eight, we could predict that in about eighteen or twenty months she would probably need dialysis—or perhaps a kidney transplant. We discussed what it would be like to live with either option, and Janice went home to talk things over with her husband. One factor she considered is that long-term dialysis is often more difficult for people with diabetes than for others, so that the complications and mortality are about doubled. After some thought she asked to be put on the waiting list for a new kidney.

Like an ever increasing number of people in her circumstances, Janice preferred transplantation to long-term dialysis. Even so, she still would require insulin therapy, and the complications of her diabetes would continue to progress. The statistics told us that in five to ten years she would have a high risk of dying from a heart attack or stroke. So when we brought up the option of a combined pancreas and kidney transplant, she said, "Let's do it."

Among its other functions, the pancreas produces insulin, which is essential for the normal metabolism of sugar. It was the failure of her pancreas at around age eleven that caused Janice's juvenile diabetes. With her consent, we put her name on the list of people waiting for pancreas *and* kidney transplantation. She began the typically long and frustrating wait for a suitable donor. During that eight-month wait, her kidney function deteriorated to the point where she required dialysis. Finally, a donor was identified, and Janice was called to the hospital for the dual transplant.

History and Current Technique

In contrast to the surgical techniques for kidney, liver, and heart transplantation—which were worked out fifteen to twenty-five years ago—the major advances in replacing the pancreas are new in the last five years. The first attempt to perform this operation on a human was undertaken in 1966 at the University of Minnesota. But progress in this field lagged well behind that of other solid organ transplants, largely because of the technical difficulties in performing this very complex surgery. Of the sixty operations tried between 1966 and 1977, only two transplanted organs functioned for more than one year. Despite research in the field, high rates of infection and blood clots in the replacement organ, along with many other problems, persisted. We seemed to be facing an insurmountable hurdle. Nevertheless, surgeons continued to look for new approaches, such as transplanting only a portion of the donor organ, or just a purified portion of the organ's cells (called *islet cells*) that produce insulin. In laboratory animals, at least, the latter approach was successful in reversing the diabetes and its complications, but uncertainty continued as to the quantity of islet cells needed for human transplantation. As research continued, new techniques were developed, and several recently reported short-term successes following islet transplantation suggest this approach may soon become the

preferred treatment. Currently, however, the most widely uti-
lized technique involves using the entire donor pancreas, along
with a small portion of its drainage system, and making a
connection with the bladder. This permits fluid from the pancreas to drain into the urine without entering the bowel, and
avoids potential infectious complications arising from microorganisms living in the intestinal tract. Also, by measuring the
acid and amylase concentrations in the urine, we have a simple
and safe way to assess the new transplant's function. For
people like Janice, with longstanding insulin-dependent diabetes, combined pancreas and kidney transplantation now
seems to provide a modest advantage over renal transplant
alone.

> Immediately after her operation, Janice had no further
> need for dialysis or insulin. For the first time in more
> than twenty years she was free of the daily injections that
> had become part of her life. "I can have blueberry pie
> without feeling guilty," she said with a smile. "That
> means for the first time since I was eleven, I don't have
> to lie to myself or my doctor when I break my diet."

Selecting Donor and Recipient

Much of what we have said already about choosing donor and
recipient for other transplant operations applies to pancreas
replacement. The recipient must be cleared for surgery and
understand the postoperative immunosuppression that will be
required. We also are concerned that the recipient not have
advanced eye or peripheral nerve degeneration, serious heart
disease, or compromise of the peripheral blood vessels. If these
conditions are advanced, the likelihood of postoperative complications, even death, is high. Before surgery, tests are completed to make certain the donor's kidney and pancreas are
functioning well. Donor and recipient are matched for blood
type, and a crossmatch is performed (see Chapter 2). Because
the number of donors is extremely limited, more extensive
matching is not generally practical. Once recipient and donor

are selected, the pancreas must be removed and promptly transported to the recipient's hospital. Because techniques for preserving the pancreas outside the body are not as advanced as for the kidney or liver, we try to complete the replacement operation within twelve to fifteen hours after the donor organ is removed.

The Operation

A successful pancreas transplant begins with meticulous care in removing the donor organ. Experience has shown that trauma to the donor pancreas is a major factor leading to complications after transplantation. Once delivered to the recipient, we attach it to his or her blood circulation by sewing the donor's portal vein and arteries (these are the same blood vessels that supply the liver) to the major leg vein and artery located in the recipient's lower abdomen. As noted already, in order to reduce the risk of a bacterial infection that might come from the bowel, the digestive drainage of the pancreas is connected to the recipient's bladder. While the insulin will flow into the bloodstream via the circulatory system, the potentially caustic digestive secretions will drain safely into the urine. The final maneuver is the removal of the donor's spleen, which was left attached to the pancreas during the procedure to encourage increased blood flow during the early rewarming period when spasm of the blood vessels would compromise the operation. The kidney operation proceeds as has been described already, usually before the pancreas procedure is begun.

After Surgery

Again, much of what goes on after transplanting both the pancreas and the kidney is the same as for replacing the kidney alone. But because blood clotting has complicated about 20 percent of pancreas transplants in the past, it is now common to administer anticoagulant medications during the first several days after surgery. This preventive measure is followed by a daily aspirin at home for the next several months.

Janice did well after her surgery. She was up and around in a few days, seemingly not fazed by postoperative pain. Within the first twenty-four hours her new pancreas was producing a self-regulating supply of insulin. Neither during nor after surgery did she require insulin. In fact, until she began eating, her blood sugar tended to be a little lower than normal, because her insulin was flowing directly into the bloodstream, rather than through the liver as is normal.

After the tyranny of injecting insulin each day and restricting her life-style, convalescing seemed a small price to pay. Her family was there too, keeping her company and encouraging her to come home soon. Now, it was time to review her medications, make plans for follow-up clinic visits, and see to the business of resuming a normal life.

For patients who have only a pancreas transplant, measuring blood sugar levels is currently the best way to assess potential organ rejection. However, a major problem with this method is that rising blood sugar, and the physical symptoms of hyperglycemia that go with it, are often not manifested until rejection is far advanced. At this late stage, it usually is not possible to reverse the rejection, because 80 or 90 percent of the insulin-producing islet cells are already permanently damaged. With combined kidney and pancreas transplantation, it is possible to monitor the kidney as an indicator of the rejection process. If at any point the assessment is in doubt, it is possible to biopsy the kidney with safety and relative ease. Unfortunately, with the techniques now available it is not judicious to do this on a regular basis for the pancreas.

In many respects, the postoperative and long-term immunosuppression regimens for dual pancreas and kidney transplants are similar to those for kidney transplants alone. We typically use a three-drug regimen, and acute rejection episodes are initially treated with an increase in the dose of steroids. If this is not successful, we add OKT3 or other medications.

One unique aspect of pancreas-kidney replacement is the use of urine tests to monitor transplant function. While for most people it is normal for the urine to be acidic, after pancreas replacement the urine is typically alkaline (basic). The amount of amylase, one of the digestive enzymes produced normally by the pancreas, found in the urine is also high. The simplest urine testing can be done at home, or at a physician's office in the community.

Results

Until recently, the results of pancreas transplantation were dismal and progress was frustratingly slow, with graft survival for the first year ranging from 3 to 40 percent. From 1978 to 1985 the results improved to about 70 percent, but only about 20 percent of recipients became insulin-independent. Recent results are far more encouraging; since 1986 about 90 percent of recipients are alive after one year, and over 50 percent are insulin-independent. These figures seem even better when they are viewed in light of the fact that many recipients were suffering from advanced complications of their diabetes. Moreover, since the one-year survival rate for diabetic patients receiving renal transplantation alone is about 90 percent, we can say that dual pancreas and kidney replacement does not present significant added risk. And in some centers the survival rate for pancreas transplantation alone is approaching that of kidney replacement, so that the future for this procedure is looking brighter every day. As of May 1990, at our hospital we have performed thirty-five dual pancreas-kidney transplants, with thirty recipients (86 percent) alive after two to forty-eight months, and twenty-eight of them completely free of the need for insulin.

It is now two years since Janice had her operation, and like most of our pancreas recipients she is enthusiastic about her new life. "I feel I can control my own destiny," she told us proudly. "All those years I accepted being dependent on insulin and restricting my diet, but I never really got used to it." So far the precise impact of the transplant on her chances of developing future complications related to diabetes, and its effect on her longevity, are still uncertain. The long-term data from laboratory animals are very encouraging, but the same information is not yet available for humans. So far, as with most pancreas recipients, the small blood vessels of her replacement kidney are not degenerating in the way we see in people with diabetes who have a kidney transplant alone. This is a very hopeful sign.

The Future

As of this writing, the International Human Pancreas Transplant Registry, which records the results of replacing the pancreas, notes that approximately 1,500 operations have been performed worldwide. Over the last three years more transplants were performed than in the previous twenty years. Survival rates for dual pancreas-kidney surgery now approach that of kidney replacement, a widely acknowledged success for modern medicine. Now that we have established that replacing the pancreas is reasonably safe, it is time to test its long-term efficacy in people who are not yet suffering kidney failure, loss of vision, and the other terrible effects of diabetes. Specific criteria for selecting individuals for the operation are still to be determined—not only because organs are in short supply, but because only about half the people with juvenile-onset diabetes go on to have the serious complications. So far, it appears that the best measure for who should be transplanted is impending kidney failure, and the best strategy is to perform the surgery before the need for dialysis. Our hope is that by performing surgery earlier we can make pancreas transplantation a method of preventing, not just treating, the complications of this terrible disease.

Transplanting the Liver

Shortly after Fred Stevens returned from a vacation in Latin America, his wife noticed a slightly yellow tint in the whites of his eyes. "You better go see the doctor," she said. He took her advice, and his family doctor made the diagnosis of viral hepatitis.

Fred's doctor was reassuring, but despite the usual medical regimen Fred's condition deteriorated. Soon he was bleeding from the gastrointestinal tract and had to be hospitalized. Despite intensive treatment, his health worsened. The bleeding would not stop. He became confused, lapsed into a coma. Early pneumonia began to develop. Tests showed that the liver was irreversibly damaged. We put Fred on the list for a new liver and waited anxiously while his coma deepened. A transplant would be his only hope.

In the last five years we have seen liver transplantation progress from a highly risky, strictly experimental procedure to one that is accepted therapy for a significant portion of the 20,000 people who otherwise would die annually in the United States from end-stage liver failure. In that short period of time, the five-year survival rate has gone from 10 to more than 50 percent, among patients who would *all* die without surgery (see Table 8.1). Only the shortage of donor organs prevents more people from benefiting from liver replacement. Liver

Table 8.1. Survival following liver transplantation.

Era	One-year survival	Five-year survival
1963–1982	30–35%	Less than 10%
1983–1990	70–80%	50–60%
No transplant	5–10%	None

Note: In less than a decade, there has been a five- to six-fold increase in long-term survival for liver transplant recipients. Without transplantation none of these individuals would have survived.

transplants from living related donors has little promise for significant impact.

History

Situated in the upper right part of the abdomen, the liver is the body's largest solid organ. Its functions are complex and numerous, including removing toxic substances from the bloodstream, metabolizing nutrients, storing energy sources, and producing enzymes and proteins essential for blood clotting. It is the failure to excrete bile, necessary to break down dietary fats, which produces the yellow jaundice that is a hallmark of liver failure.

Fortunately, the liver has a remarkable capacity to regenerate after most illnesses, so the story of Fred Stevens is a rather unusual one. In some instances, however, the liver becomes irreversibly damaged due to inherited abnormalities, excess alcohol or drug intake, cancer, or the infectious viruses that cause hepatitis. The liver develops scarring (termed *cirrhosis*), leading to potentially fatal complications, such as bleeding, infection, and the build-up of toxic waste products. The only life-saving option at this point is removing the diseased liver and transplanting a healthy organ in its place.

> While we waited for an organ, Fred's coma deepened to the point where we had to assist his breathing by machine. As the toxic waste products built up in his bloodstream, he began to have seizures, which required extensive intravenous medications. Even with that treatment, we worried that he might be suffering irreversible brain damage. And, because his blood was not clotting normally, he was bleeding from the gastrointestinal tract, as well as from the places where we had to place his IVs. Just as his death seemed imminent, we found a donor. But Fred was so ill that we worried, as we sped him to the operating room, that even a new liver might not save him.

The surgical techniques for replacing the liver in humans

were developed more than thirty years ago by teams working independently in Boston and Denver. But it was not until 1963 that a hospital team led by Dr. Thomas Starzl at the University of Colorado actually attempted the operation. Over the next four years, efforts to accomplish this formidable task produced no long-term success. It was not until 1967 that the same University of Colorado group performed a transplant that survived for a year—for a recipient who later died of a recurrence of the liver cancer for which she had originally been treated. Despite this modest success, because of limitations in both immunosuppression and surgical technique, extremely high rates of complications and death plagued the field. In contrast to the enormous success being enjoyed in kidney transplantation, it seemed that liver replacement might be an unattainable goal. As a result, except for programs lead by Starzl in Denver and Sir Roy Calne in Cambridge, England, over the next fifteen years physicians called a moratorium on liver transplantation.

At the beginning of the 1980s the almost simultaneous introduction of cyclosporine in England and monoclonal antibodies in Boston ushered in a new era for liver transplantation. With markedly improved results being realized in kidney transplants, we now felt it was time to try liver replacement again. Soon, the one-year survival rate doubled. Stimulated by this encouraging change in outcome, in 1983 a Consensus Development Conference on Liver Transplantation was convened at the National Institutes of Health in Washington, D.C. The participants concluded appropriately that liver transplantation was no longer an experimental procedure, but now a true therapeutic approach for a variety of irreversible liver diseases. This determination mandated a much broader application of the procedure, so that over the next seven years more than seventy centers in North America, and thirty in Europe, became established to perform liver transplants.

The Liver Transplant Candidate

At age sixty-one Fred was considerably older than most liver transplant recipients, although with each year of added success we are relaxing the age requirement. Certainly he had the highest of medical priorities. So when the donor organ became available we did not hesitate.

Since he was so near death, we began the operation at 4 A.M., as soon as the donor organ arrived. Seven and a half hours later the operation was complete. Fred's recovery was swift. Although he needed the mechanical ventilator for his breathing and intravenous antibiotics for his pneumonia, he was awake, no longer in a coma, within twelve hours of receiving the new liver. In addition, the bleeding stopped. We had literally been pouring blood into him, and now that was not needed. It would still take another two weeks to wean him from the mechanical breathing machine and begin his physical rehabilitation program. Nevertheless, it was a recovery hard for even us to believe. His family was ecstatic.

Unfortunately, selecting a liver recipient from the large population of candidates needing a transplant involves excluding some individuals. For the most part, they are people who are too ill to benefit from surgery. Today, many of the criteria used to restrict selection of candidates—such as age—are being relaxed, as proficiency in performing the procedure improves. The oldest person transplanted so far was seventy-seven, an age unheard of only a few years ago. Active cancer does remain an important reason for exclusion unless we can be certain to remove all traces of it. Otherwise, although survival is excellent in the immediate postoperative period, over the long term there is a high risk that the cancer will recur. Part of the pretransplant evaluation, therefore, is extensive testing to rule out a hidden cancer that would not be fully eliminated by removing the diseased liver. Other reasons for exclusion are uncontrollable infection outside the liver or life-threatening heart or lung disease. Currently active drug or alcohol addiction is another reason for excluding a candidate, since experience has shown that persons with active substance-abuse problems have a high likelihood of failing to follow their immunosuppressive medication regimen. On the other hand, people who demonstrate the ability to control an earlier addiction should be accepted as candidates, since their results are as good as those for the general population.

With improving success in transplanting the liver, the goal now is to identify suitable candidates *early*, before their disease is far advanced. In this sense, the story of our sixty-one-year-old recipient is a bit unusual. Nowadays, we like to provide organ replacement before there are major complications, and before patients undergo major operations or other invasive procedures. Operating relatively early avoids problems that complicate surgery later on. The desire to balance early transplantation with the need to provide the gift of life for seriously ill people sometimes presents difficult ethical problems in allocating organs.

Matching Donor and Recipient

Usually the donor is a young man or woman who has suffered brain death as a result of an accident or a stroke. With the support of a mechanical breathing apparatus, the vital major organs are maintained in a healthy state until they can be used for transplantation. For liver replacement, matching blood group is desirable, but not absolutely necessary. While it increases somewhat the likelihood of a successful transplant, the desperate need of a mortally ill person is more important than the blood group match. As in heart and lung transplantation, we try to match donor and recipient for size. The surgery is easier to perform when the donor is the same size as or slightly smaller than the recipient. This is particularly important when transplanting a liver into a small child. Since there are many more needy children than available organs, a new approach is to transplant a *segment* of an adult liver, usually from a cadaveric donor but, in rare instances, from a living relative. If this strategy works for long-term survival, it will be a major advance for both children and adults, making it possible to provide liver replacement for two patients from a single cadaveric donor. With current technologic advances, we now can preserve the liver for about twenty-four hours after it is removed from the donor's circulation. While this is sufficient time to proceed with tissue matching, in almost all instances the urgent medical need of the recipient precludes this approach.

The Operation

Most of the surgical techniques for transplanting the liver were perfected about twenty-five years ago. The diseased liver is removed and the donor organ is placed into the right upper abdomen. While this may sound relatively easy, the surgery actually is quite demanding, requiring from six to eighteen hours. At least three surgeons, two anesthetists, and a half-dozen nurses are needed during the procedure. The diseased liver must be disconnected from four major blood vessels, and the duct that carries bile from the liver to the intestines must be severed from the bowel. Since all the major veins carrying blood from the lower body enter the liver, this blood flow is necessarily interrupted during the operation. Not all recipients would be able to tolerate this stress, so a significant advance has been to develop a special pump, related to the heart-lung machine described in Chapter 7. With this machine, blood flows in an alternative loop from the lower body and intestines back to the heart, thereby bypassing the surgical field. Especially for very ill people, this new technique seems to be helpful. Completing the transplant requires reattaching the major blood vessels and bile duct. The amount of blood lost often is several times the recipient's entire blood volume. The exact quantity involved must be assessed very carefully, so that the amount replaced matches closely the amount that was lost. This is one of the essential tasks of the anesthesiology team. Recently, there have been important steps forward in learning to recover and reintroduce into circulation the patient's own blood that is shed into the operative field.

Once the blood vessels are reconnected and the occluding clamps are released, blood begins to flow through the donor organ. At this point the pale donor organ begins to turn pink and to produce bile and the body's natural clotting factors. If there is profuse abnormal bleeding, it soon abates. If the patient was in a coma, after awakening from anesthesia, the mind will be clearing. To see this phenomenon is to appreciate the gift of life.

Recovery

During the initial period after liver transplantation, the care is more complicated than after kidney or pancreas surgery. In large part, this is because of the recipient's usually precarious preoperative medical condition. In addition, the long and arduous surgery, with the massive loss of fluid and blood, takes its toll. At first, all new recipients go to the intensive care unit and breathe on a respirator. If all goes well, the breathing machine can be gradually phased out over twenty-four to forty-eight hours. However, it is not unusual to need assistance with breathing for a longer period.

It is now time to begin to fine tune the immunosuppressive medications. If kidney function is compromised, as it often is, it may be necessary to substitute anti-lymphocyte globulin or OKT3 for cyclosporine (see Chapter 3). Since the medications reduce resistance to infection, intensive respiratory therapy is required to prevent, or treat, lung infection.

It seemed like clear sailing for the first week. With the combination of the antibiotics and respiratory treatments, Fred's pneumonia cleared. His kidneys began working. His spirits improved. The first setback came about one week after surgery, when blood tests revealed that his liver function was declining. Experience told us that Fred was suffering his first rejection episode. Because he still had some evidence of the pneumonia, we were reluctant to increase the dose of steroids, which might exacerbate the infection. So we gave him intravenous doses of OKT3, which is more selective than steroids in altering the immune barrier. Fortunately, the rejection seemed to reverse, and over approximately ten days his liver function returned to normal.

Early on, the most hopeful sign of a successful transplant is improving liver function. Most initial episodes of rejection can be treated by altering the medical regimen, so that only about 10 percent of recipients require immediate retransplantation.

After three to ten days in intensive care, the recipient spends another two to four weeks convalescing in the transplant unit before discharge. During this time, we watch closely for signs of rejection, such as fever, back pain, jaundice, fluid accumulating in the abdomen, and laboratory evidence of diminishing liver function. Like Fred, about half of all recipients will have at least one episode of acute rejection. With increased immunosuppression, these episodes usually are reversed. We also emphasize aggressive nutritional and physical rehabilitation. Most people resume eating during the first week after surgery, but after months of malnourishment it may also be helpful to take supplemental nutrition via a feeding tube placed into the stomach through the nose (a nasogastric tube). Along with the inactivity and poor nutrition of liver failure inevitably comes loss of muscle mass and physical stamina. Therefore, the postoperative convalescing period involves intensive physical therapy and personal effort to get back in shape.

During the first months after discharge from the hospital, most recipients return to the transplant unit once or twice a week for follow-up visits. It is also important to come to the hospital for a regular program of physical rehabilitation. For people not living near the transplant center, that usually means renting an apartment. During medical visits we carefully assess liver function, regulate the medications, and look for potential occult (silent) infections. While a liver recipient, like any other transplant recipient, must take immunosuppressive medicines for the rest of his or her life, fortunately the dose needed to maintain the new organ diminishes over time. As the risks of infection and rejection decline, the frequency of follow-up visits also goes down. By eight to ten weeks after surgery most people are at home, visiting their family physician or community liver specialist for follow-up medical care.

Despite having been perhaps only a precious few hours from death, Fred recovered splendidly. On the thirty-third day after surgery he left the hospital for a nearby apartment to continue outpatient physical therapy and clinic visits. Soon, he was home, getting his strength back and enjoying a new perspective on life. By six months following transplantation he was back teaching and defeating his usual tennis opponents. Now, four years after his operation, at age sixty-five, Fred's step is lively, and he enjoys robust health.

Today and Tomorrow

The expected five-year survival rate for liver transplantation is now more than 50 percent. Once the vulnerable early period of about three months passes, almost all recipients enjoy excellent recovery to a full, active life. In children, this includes returning to good physical health and resuming normal growth and development. In addition, youngsters get back their emotional sense of well-being, including returning almost immediately to their expected performance at school. Most adults find they can go back to work, and so far about 80 percent have chosen to do so. They tell us that they feel well, and have a new sense of mental clarity and stamina on the job.

Since the experience with improved survival and rehabilitation is so new, it is difficult to know with certainty the true picture for the long term. A few patients who received the early transplants are still alive after twenty years. With continued advances in immunosuppressive therapy, our hope is that their experience will become the rule more than the exception.

With long-term survival a reality, replacing the liver moves from an experimental treatment to an accepted medical therapy. As a consequence, other factors limiting its widespread application must be addressed. The first is the cost, which typically runs between $100,000 and $200,000, although it can be even greater. While these numbers certainly are daunting, they probably do not exceed the cost of caring for a chronically ill person suffering from advanced liver disease. The cost of the person's disability, including loss of income, medications, hospitalizations, palliative surgical treatments, and predictably terminal care, often equals or exceeds this amount. But virtually all of these patients die of their disease. It thus seems to us that liver transplantation is cost-effective, as well as the logical and humane thing to do.

The second major obstacle limiting more widespread liver transplantation is an inadequate supply of donor organs. Currently, too many people die while waiting for a new liver. It is estimated that about 18,000 people die each year who could be suitable donors. But for a variety of reasons we are able to obtain organs in only about 20 percent of these deaths. A vital national resource is being underutilized. Clearly, new approaches are needed to increase the number of organs available for transplantation, and to improve the network by which they are allocated. How we overcome the economic, ethical, and logistical problems will thus determine how far and how fast we can extend the benefits of liver transplantation to needy people. Technology will also play a role, particularly if non-human donor organs and better immunosuppressives can be developed. Such advances not only would make the procedure available to more recipients but might make it less expensive. Yet, with these caveats said, it still is fair to say that liver transplantation has come of age, providing hope and a new life to patients who only a few years ago would have died from end-stage liver disease.

9

Bone Marrow Transplantation

When we first met Per Lindstrom, he was thirty-one years old, married, with a beautiful two-year-old son. Born in Denmark, but firmly ensconced in his American life, Per seemed to be the picture of Nordic health: tall, blond, trim, and outdoorsy. "Until just a few weeks ago I thought my life was perfect," he said. "I felt fine. In fact I had never felt better." But he told us of a sudden, frightening turnaround in his health.

A few months earlier, he had noticed that he was tiring easily. He just could not put in a full day at the office. For a few weeks the fatigue persisted, and then he sensed a new ache under his rib cage on the left side. Soon he was coughing a lot, and the pain in his side would double him over. Then his vision began to blur. What Per had thought was just a lingering virus now prompted an emergency visit to his family doctor.

Per's doctor quickly pinpointed an enlarged spleen as the cause of the pain on his left side. He also found the potential cause of the blurred vision: small hemorrhages on the surface of the retina at the back of the eye. The findings were disturbing. Retinal hemorrhage in a young man who does not have diabetes is extremely rare. Per's doctor drew some blood for laboratory analysis and sent him to see an ophthalmologist (a physician who specializes in eye disorders).

The blood tests revealed a very high white blood cell count of 200,000 and anemia. The normal white cell count is somewhere between 4,000 and 10,000; the anemia was occurring because the abnormal white cells were crowding out his normal red blood cells. Moreover, when examined under the microscope, his white blood cells were markedly irregular in their shape and overall appearance. These were all ominous signs, and Per was referred to the Brigham and Women's Hospital for further evaluation.[1]

A biopsy of Per's bone marrow confirmed the diagnosis of chronic myelogenous leukemia, or CML, which his family doctor had strongly suspected. We informed Per that drug treatments, called chemotherapy, were available to control his leukemia for a time, but that they were unlikely to cure it. We told him it might be a year, or it might be three to five years, but his leukemia would eventually progress. It would ultimately be fatal.

But there was another option: bone marrow transplantation, a new and risky technique offering the hope of curing his otherwise incurable disease. It did not take Per long to make his decision. "I want the transplant," he said firmly.

During the 1950s, laboratory scientists first observed that high doses of radiation would destroy the bone marrow of mice and kill them within a few weeks. In confirming what already had been noted at the bombings of Hiroshima and Nagasaki, this finding in itself was not particularly surprising. What was remarkable was that the mice could be saved, if after the potentially lethal radiation they were given an injection of replacement bone marrow from a genetically identical mouse.

1. In this chapter, mentions of "our" hospital refer to Brigham and Women's.

Miraculously, the new bone marrow would reconstitute the irradiated marrow, thereby rebuilding the mouse's destroyed immune system.

Meanwhile, another scientific breakthrough was in progress. We began to develop skill in chemotherapy, the use of anticancer drugs, along with radiation, to treat malignancies of the blood-forming system (such as leukemia and lymphoma). Unfortunately, the newly emerging and very potent anticancer treatments frequently also caused irreversible damage to the bone marrow. So, while it was possible to eradicate the cancer, in the process we also would be dealing a fatal blow to the immune system.

An obvious approach was to apply to people the new technique learned in mice. Why not first kill the cancer cells and then replace the destroyed bone marrow with new, healthy marrow via a bone marrow transplant? By the late 1950s and early 1960s, approximately 200 bone marrow transplants had been performed around the world. But the initial results were dismal, as fatal complications inevitably arose during the transplant process. Most significantly, the new bone marrow attacked the body's vital organs, a process known as graft-versus-host disease or GVH. Tragically, the patients who survived the chemotherapy and radiation perished from the transplant itself. It soon was clear that finding a perfect match between donor and recipient was even more critical in bone marrow transplantation (BMT) than in solid organ replacement. And because the results of the first bone marrow transplants were so poor, virtually all major medical centers gave up on the idea.

During the 1970s several major breakthroughs occurred in the field of immunology that revived interest in BMT. By far the most significant was learning to more accurately define an individual's histocompatibility leukocyte antigens, or HLA type (see Chapter 3). Produced normally by all cells of the body, HLA is a collection of proteins that reside on the surface of these cells. Passed down genetically at the time of conception from parents to offspring, HLA works like an immunologic fingerprint that marks each cell. The principal player in the system is the T cell, a type of white blood cell whose job it is to travel through the bloodstream inspecting for foreign cells. The T cell is the immune system's tireless policeman, continually searching for cells that do not have the correct markings. When an inspector T cell sees a cell whose fingerprint matches his own, he lets it pass unharmed; if, on the other hand, he finds a cell—a bacterium or fungus, for instance—that does not have the right markings, he labels it foreign and targets it for destruction. This constant vigilance is termed immune surveillance.

However, the immune surveillance system was until recently the bane of bone marrow transplantation. In developing accurate laboratory tests to describe an individual's HLA type, we became capable of detecting donor bone marrow that would attack the recipient, thus causing GVH. Rather quickly we also discovered that a good HLA match is most readily found among siblings. Thus, the majority of the approximately 20,000 bone marrow transplants that have been performed to date in the United States have relied on finding a close family member to be the donor. Additionally, about 100,000 people around the world have been HLA typed, and this information has been stored in a computer, thereby creating a bank at which people who do not have an HLA-identical family member can search for a potentially suitable bone marrow donor. More will be said about this aspect of BMT later in this chapter.

In addition to the improvement in our ability to make a good match between donor and recipient, over the last two decades bone marrow transplantation has benefited from dramatic medical advances in the fields of chemotherapy, radiation, antibiotic therapy, and powerful radiological and diagnostic testing. As a result, BMT is now the treatment of choice for certain types of leukemia (such as chronic myelogenous leukemia, or CML), aplastic anemia (when the bone marrow fails), and a rather rare disorder of unknown cause called severe combined childhood immune deficiency syndrome. In addition, there is growing evidence that BMT may be useful in some forms of lymphoma. Relapsed acute leukemia and testicular cancer may also be treatable with BMT. There now are at least seventy-five medical centers in the United States, Canada, and Europe performing bone marrow transplants, serving two to three thousand recipients annually. Currently, most insurance companies cover bone marrow transplantation for the above-mentioned conditions, although at least one state—Oregon—does not cover this service. More experimental uses of BMT, such as in treating solid tumors (such as advanced breast and testicular cancer or sarcomas), may not, however, be funded by commercial insurance.

The Organ

Unlike the kidneys, lungs, heart, liver, and pancreas, bone marrow is a liquid, not a solid, organ. Nevertheless, we should think of it as just like any other organ, capable of being transplanted from a donor to a recipient. Residing in the cavities of the body's large bones, such as the spine, breastbone, pelvis, and leg bones, the marrow is a factory whose principal workers are millions of floating master cells. Known also as stem cells, they churn out offspring that will mature into the billions of red blood cells, white blood cells, and platelets that populate the bloodstream.

Of the three principal types of mature cells in the bloodstream, the red cells, or erythrocytes, work to transport oxygen from the lungs to the tissues. While circulating in the bloodstream, these tiny, disc-shaped forms are actually blue in color, turning red only when exposed to oxygen in the lung. A deficiency of these cells produces anemia, whose symptoms include easy fatigue, generalized weakness, skin pallor, and sometimes rapid heart rate and breathing rate—the symptoms Per Lindstrom first noted as a sign of his developing leukemia. Laboratory assessment of anemia is accomplished in a number of ways, including by obtaining a small sample of blood and measuring the concentration of *hematocrit* (the percentage of red cells in a standardized volume of blood) or *hemoglobin* (the oxygen-carrying capacity). If these numbers are low one is likely to be anemic. It should be emphasized that anemia is a symptom with many underlying causes: if the hematocrit or hemoglobin is low, it is important to determine the basic cause of the problem and direct treatment as specifically as possible.

The white blood cells are the journeymen of the immune system, serving to both fight infection and prevent cancer. Unlike the red cells, white cells come in a number of different types, including T cells (important in graft-versus-host disease), B cells, "killer" cells, and polymorphonuclear cells, nicknamed polys. The polys are the pus-fighting cells, critical to protecting the body from the billions of potentially infectious organisms that come in contact with us each day. As we shall see later, after bone marrow transplantation we carefully monitor the poly count, as it provides a vital index of the immune system's recovery.

Finally, there are the platelets, the smallest of the three principal types of blood cells, which function as floating bandages to prevent abnormal or excess bleeding. When bleeding begins, platelets congregate at the site of injury and plug the hole. Low platelet levels in the circulating bloodstream, a condition known as *thrombocytopenia*, can lead to serious abnormal bleeding. Unfortunately, platelets also may sometimes congregate in unwanted places, clogging an artery and thereby producing a heart attack or stroke.

If you look at a small section of healthy marrow under the microscope, you see a few mature blood cells, along with many active master cells interspersed within a supporting scaffolding of fibrous tissue and fat. In someone who has leukemia, all you see are the abnormal leukemic cells; in aplastic anemia, another condition potentially treatable with BMT, you see pretty much only the scaffolding. As we discuss further on, in either case the purpose of the transplant is to repopulate the factory with healthy stem cells that will migrate to the scaffolding, take hold, and begin to grow and multiply like normal bone marrow. Indeed, before administering the new marrow we filter out the mature red cells and platelets, leaving a cream-colored mixture whose most important constituent is the donor's stem cells. Once the healthy marrow takes hold, it will continue to be the future source for replenishing all essential blood lines for a lifetime.

The BMT Option

In solid organ transplantation, we usually are replacing the diseased organ because it can no longer maintain life without extraordinary medical support. The rationale for bone marrow transplantation is, perhaps, a bit more complex, in that there are now three major indications for undergoing the procedure.

Leukemia

Probably the most common reason we perform BMT is leukemia, the medical term for cancer of the blood-forming cells. There are a number of different leukemias, each type affecting a different master cell line, and each having a different prognosis. In the leukemias, the marrow and bloodstream are crowded with very high levels of abnormal white blood cells, which sooner or later overwhelm the normal cells. The result is anemia, abnormal bleeding, and susceptibility to serious infection. Leukemia is often rapidly fatal if not treated. Fortunately, many children and some adults now can be cured of leukemia with aggressive chemotherapy. There are, however, some patients who cannot be cured with the drug therapies now available. For these people, bone marrow transplantation offers the best chance for cure.

When Per Lindstrom came to our hospital he was facing an uncertain but undoubtedly rather circumscribed future. His type of leukemia, CML, could be held at bay at most for six or seven years—and that was a long shot— with current medical therapy. We told him that with bone marrow transplantation there was a chance his disease could be cured. But it might not work, and there might be complications.

Per asked about the complications and the chances. We gave him some rough estimates. "Let's say we have a hundred people with leukemia like yours. If we do BMT, about fifteen or twenty will not be cured of their cancer. Another fifteen or twenty, let's say, will get a fatal complication of their transplant, and another twenty or twenty-five will have very bad graft-versus-host disease. That leaves about thirty-five who will be fully cured, at least as far as we know right now."

The conversation stopped for these facts to settle in. "That means," we summarized, "you have about a 30 percent chance that you'll have no serious, lingering side-effects from your transplant, your cancer will be cured, and you won't need to take drugs or have other treatments. It's not an easy choice, but it's where things currently stand."

Thus, while we could offer a potential cure for Per's otherwise fatal disease, we still had a rather long way to go before we could promise him the relatively certain success of, for instance, a kidney transplant. In that procedure, out of a hundred people transplanted, about ninety would probably be living with their new organ after the first year, and seventy-five would go on for an even longer time—taking immunosuppressive drugs, of course, but nevertheless living productive, fairly average lives.

Bone Marrow Failure

The second indication for bone marrow transplantation is marrow failure occurring independently of an underlying cancer. The conditions that cause the bone marrow to stop producing blood cells are, fortunately, relatively uncommon. Some babies, for instance, are born without normally functioning stem cells, probably as a result of a genetic abnormality. If the fetus fails to develop normal red blood cells it will not mature in the uterus and will probably never grow to term. On the other hand, if the fetus does not develop normal immune defenses, it can still mature in the protected environment of the womb. Once delivered, however, the infant becomes susceptible to infectious agents. After birth, these youngsters become sickly and may require bone marrow transplantation as a life-saving measure.

Some people—again fortunately not very many—lose their master cells later in childhood or adulthood. Some of these situations are thought to be the result of an autoimmune process, such as rheumatoid arthritis, in which the body's T cells erroneously decide that its own stem cells are foreign. Going haywire in this way, the body's immune system attacks the marrow, killing off the master cells. There are also some viral infections, as well as toxic drugs and chemicals, that may destroy the stem cells. Regardless of whether one or all three of the master cell lines are being affected, or what the underlying cause of the illness is, BMT is a potentially life-saving way to replace depleted marrow.

Cancer

Bone marrow transplantation is now being employed with increasing frequency for the treatment of cancers other than leukemia. The need for BMT typically arises when the marrow is irreversibly damaged by aggressive, potentially life-saving, cancer therapy. In these instances, we have been forced to push chemotherapeutic doses higher and higher in an effort to cure a tumor not responding to more standard treatment. While we may succeed in reducing dramatically—even eradicating—the cancer, in the process we also destroy the normal bone marrow. One recent approach to this problem is to obtain and store the patient's own marrow before initiating the high doses of anticancer drugs. Once the chemotherapy is finished, we transplant his or her marrow back in an autologous (from *auto*, self) transplant.

Robert Darnell is an avid fly fisherman we recently treated after an eight-year battle with Hodgkin's disease. On three occasions his disease relapsed, despite treatment that often is successful in curing his type of cancer. Each time it came back, we administered higher doses of chemotherapy and radiation. Now it was recurring for the third time, and his best chance for a cure was an even higher dose of drugs. This time the treatment was very likely to do severe damage to his bone marrow.

On the positive side, his bone marrow was still normal. So before we began the high-dose regimen we removed, froze, and stored some of his normal marrow to transplant back into him later. "Once we finish the chemotherapy," we told him, "and see that your Hodgkin's is arrested, we'll reintroduce the stored bone marrow. If all goes well you may be cured."

Bob is now back to his family and his fishing, doing well without any evidence of his cancer. After several years of disability, he has returned to work. Whenever he hears that one of us is going on vacation, he asks if we know of a good fishing stream in the vicinity. Ever since contracting cancer he's been acutely aware of how fragile life is. He's developed a new attitude about things: no longer the hard-driving executive, he tries to carry on his days doing what he wants to do.

Before the Transplant

In order to know whether BMT is advisable for any given patient, we begin with a battery of tests to assess heart, lung, kidney, and liver function. The simplest of these involve obtaining urine and blood samples, a chest X-ray, and an electrocardiogram (EKG). If the results indicate that the person is likely to withstand the rigors of transplantation, the potential recipient and family meet with the social workers and nurses on our team, who will assist them during the five-week transplant hospitalization. In addition, we schedule an examination with our dentist, who is especially knowledgeable about the oral hygiene problems that can arise during BMT. The dental evaluation involves a complete oral examination, prophylaxis (cleaning), and treatment of caries (cavities) or other areas that might be potential sites for infection. Finally, if an *allogenic* transplant is to be performed—that is, a transplant from sibling to sibling—arrangements are made to collect the donor marrow just before the anticipated date of the transplant. Because bone marrow is taken from a living donor, the procedure, unlike a heart of liver transplant, can be scheduled weeks in advance. Preparations must be made for the donor to travel to our hospital, be tested, undergo the donor operation and, if necessary, be lodged. While bone marrow can theoretically be frozen, stored, and thawed for subsequent transplantation, we prefer to have the donor come to our hospital. If for some reason frozen marrow could not be used after being thawed, there would be a terrible problem because the recipient would have already undergone bone marrow *ablation*, which destroys normal immune system function (see below for more about ablation). On the other hand, for patients who are receiving their own bone marrow, it is relatively safe and easy to freeze and store the marrow and transplant it many months later.

Finding a Match

We began looking for a potential bone marrow donor among Per's brothers, who were living in Denmark. After a check at a hospital near Copenhagen, blood samples from one brother were sent to our hospital, where we analyzed the HLA type. The brother's blood checked out on the first, serologic test. Now there was the even more sensitive proliferative match to perform. In this test we mixed donor and recipient's lymphocytes to see if the cells would become "excited." If, when mingled in the test container, the cells became stimulated and began dividing rapidly, we would expect poor results if we tried to do the transplant. Fortunately, Per's brother's blood sample passed the test. We had a match.

Per then contacted his brother in Denmark, making arrangements for him to fly to the United States to donate his bone marrow. The day after his arrival, the brother found himself at our hospital, getting a basic physical exam and a few more tests. He passed these tests too, and the next morning he was in the operating room having his marrow harvested.

The procedure was in no way as gruesome as it might sound. We can use either general anesthesia—where the donor is fully asleep—or a spinal anesthetic that numbs the lower half of the body. Per's brother chose the spinal. Next, we thoroughly cleaned the skin over his hips, lower back, and buttocks with a sterilizing solution. To accomplish the harvest, we inserted a number of sturdy needles into the pelvis and by gentle suctioning withdrew approximately one quart of red, slightly gelatinous, healthy bone marrow. The entire procedure took a little over an hour. After the harvest he went to the recovery room, and the next morning he was discharged.

After a few days with sore buttocks, the only remaining sign of the harvesting procedure was a few small puncture marks where the needles had pierced the skin. There would be no permanent, unsightly scars, and serious side-effects are almost unheard of. Perhaps the hardest part for Per's brother was waiting to see if the transplant would work.

Per Lindstrom was fortunate in that he had a sibling available to provide a donor match. There are others who are not so lucky. For these patients we must find a donor who is unrelated. We now have a computer catalogue of the name, address, and HLA type of everyone who gives bone marrow. Since bone marrow, unlike a kidney or a heart, grows back after the harvest, it is possible for one donor to give the gift of healthy marrow to more than one recipient. So, if there is no family member available for a needy recipient, we check the computer for a potential match.

The cost of finding a donor through the computer registry

can be considerable. While the initial HLA screen costs only about $500, we still must perform the more sensitive tests that require mixing in a test tube fresh blood samples from donor and recipient. If, for instance, the computer comes up with ten potential matches, we must fly samples of blood from each of these potential donors to a central laboratory where they can be tested against the recipient's blood. The cost for screening ten potential matches is approximately $10,000, and if the test fails on all of the samples we must start over. With 20,000 or so possible HLA types, there is never a guarantee we will be successful. Finally, even if one of the matches works, there is still no certainty that the donor will be available to come to the recipient's hospital and provide the marrow.

Inevitably, there are times when we cannot find a match among our registry of current names. It turns out, however, that HLA is not the sole factor in finding a suitable match. There are other genes that are important in making bone marrow compatible for transplantation. A family member—other than a sibling—can thus occasionally provide the replacement marrow. Among groups that have been closely interrelated over the centuries, such as Jews of Eastern European ancestry, there is a higher likelihood than in the general population of finding a match among parents, aunts, or uncles. This is still a desperate measure, however, without a high likelihood of success.

Yet another possibility is trying the bone marrow from an unrelated person who is not a perfect HLA match. Currently, we perform kidney and, especially, heart and liver transplants, when the match is not perfect. In BMT, however, we usually pay a heavy price in graft-versus-host disease when the match is not optimal. Nevertheless, some medical centers at this time do transplant mismatched bone marrow. This is done only when all else fails, because the near-term likelihood of death following transplantation, which is 10 to 15 percent with matched marrow, rises to 40 or 50 percent with unmatched marrow. And some of the recipients who survive will go on to develop graft-versus-host disease over the longer term.

There is currently one new, although highly experimental, possibility when no match can be found. It is called *purging*, and involves harvesting a patient's own diseased marrow and then using sophisticated laboratory techniques to kill only the leukemic cells, leaving the normal cells. The remaining treated marrow is frozen, the patient undergoes ablation, and the treated marrow is then thawed and transplanted. This technique is risky, and there are only a very few medical centers where it is performed.

Ablation

It was about six months after his leukemia was first diagnosed that Per entered the hospital to have his bone marrow transplant. The first step was to surgically implant a special catheter, called a Hickman, that would provide access to the bloodstream for administering medications and fluids. To accomplish this, we made a small incision in the skin near the nipple and threaded a catheter into the vein just under the collarbone.

With the Hickman in place we were ready to begin ablation of Per's bone marrow. Per was admitted onto the special bone marrow transplant floor, where all of the rooms are singles with ventilating systems that filter and sterilize the air. Everything in the room, including the food brought in, is also cleaned and sterilized to reduce the risk of infection. There also are comforts not usually expected in a hospital room: a television with a VCR, an exercise bike. Over the next five days we administered very high doses of chemotherapy and radiation that killed all of the cells in Per's bone marrow.

Like all patients undergoing ablation, Per was nauseated and lost his appetite. We gave him antinausea drugs, which minimized the unpleasant symptoms but also made him drowsy. He slept through most of the first few days of the ablation, a not altogether unpleasant side-effect for someone bored by the confinement of a

hospital room. The three-day course of total-body irradiation we added to the drug regimen was entirely painless,
each session lasting only fifteen minutes twice a day in
the radiotherapy suite of the hospital. But like the drugs,
the radiation is toxic, adding to the nausea and fatigue,
while also producing hair loss.

Because ablation destroys the normal master cells as well
as the diseased leukemic cells, the body's resources of red and
white blood cells and platelets drop rapidly. It is at this time
that the patient's immune system weakens. We now take even
more care to maintain the patient's personal hygiene, as well
as the cleanliness of the hospital room and the food. The
number of medical professionals who come in contact with the
patient is restricted, and they enter the room only after scrubbing and donning gowns and face masks. The sterile precautions are much like those of the operating room. After
scrubbing, family members can visit, but no one with a cold
or other illness is permitted to enter the room.

Transplantation

For the most part, Per sailed through his ablation. He
was tired, and developed some mouth sores, but these
side-effects were not unusual. We took frequent blood
tests and let him know how things were progressing. By
the time the ablation was over Per's leukemia was gone,
but so was his immune system.

   After seven days of ablation chemotherapy and radiation, it was time for Per to receive his brother's bone
marrow. Unlike the complicated surgery required in solid
organ replacement, the bone marrow transplant is simple—in many ways it is anticlimactic. Delivered to Per's
sterile room, the cream-colored fluid arrived in the kind
of plastic bag we also use for an ordinary blood transfusion. Per watched television while we dripped about a

quart of the replacement marrow into his bloodstream through the Hickman catheter. It took about thirty minutes. Once in the body, the master cells slowly migrated to his bone marrow cavity, where they implanted onto the scaffolding, began to divide, and gradually started the process of replenishing his depleted blood cells.

With ablation and transplantation completed, it is time to obtain daily blood samples to check for possible damage to the liver, heart, or lungs. Infection is also a major threat. Indeed Per, like most recipients, developed a fever that lasted for days. We administered intravenous antibiotics, hoping to suppress any possible underlying infectious agent. Using the daily blood samples, we also monitored the growth and development of his replacement marrow. Although each recipient is somewhat different, evidence that the transplant is succeeding in taking hold—a process called *engraftment*—typically can be seen sometime between seven and fourteen days after transplantation. And while the appearance of the first new, mature white cells—called *leukocytes*—is encouraging, it will still be a few more weeks before there are enough of them to protect the body from infection.

If the transplant is going well, sometime between the twenty-first and thirty-fifth days after the infusion of new marrow the patient's poly count or ANC (absolute neutrophil count) reaches 500. That means we can stop the antibiotics and slacken the strict rules for isolation. For the first time in five or six weeks, the recipient is allowed to leave the special room. Now, after a month or more of being bed-bound, it is time for the patient to work on physical conditioning. There are daily sessions in physical therapy, along with walking and, if the patient can tolerate it, working out on the stationary bicycle.

We watched for signs of infection while Per worked on improving his overall fitness. He walked around the BMT unit and rode the stationary bicycle for thirty-minute workouts. About twenty days after receiving his brother's bone marrow the differences were noticeable: his strength and appetite were coming back and the mouth sores he had developed during the chemotherapy were virtually healed. His fever was gone also, so we stopped the antibiotics.

At this point Per was nearing discharge; it was time to provide instruction as to what should and should not be done at home. Our dieticians discussed nutrition, while the entire team instructed Per and his wife on the signs and symptoms of graft-versus-host disease. It is absolutely essential that once discharged from the hospital, a person who has received an allogenic transplant be able to recognize these signs at the earliest possible moment.

Graft-Versus-Host Disease

Graft-versus-host disease (GVH) occurs when the newly transplanted immune system attacks the tissues and organs of the recipient. Potentially fatal, GVH is perhaps the most feared untoward outcome of bone marrow transplantation.

Normally, our T lymphocytes and other cells bear the same "fingerprints." As the T cells circulate through the body performing their customary cross-checking surveillance, they pass these other cells without activating the immune system's rejection process. But, even with our best efforts at HLA typing, the new transplant may not be a perfect immunological match. So when the newly manufactured T cells pass by the cells of the skin and the intestinal lining, for instance, they may stop and become activated. Secreting chemicals that attract other cells, they initiate an inflammatory reaction that is the earliest event in graft-versus-host disease.

We say that GVH is *acute* when it occurs during the first hundred days after transplantation, while it is *chronic* if it occurs later. Acute graft-versus-host disease may appear with many different signs and symptoms, but most commonly arises approximately three to five weeks after transplantation as rash, fever, and/or diarrhea. Sometimes there are liver abnormalities, but these usually are detected only by a blood test. Typically, the first signs of GVH are relatively mild, but if not treated properly the underlying rejection can progress to be serious or even fatal. Like most of our colleagues working at other transplant facilities, we favor obtaining a biopsy of skin, colon, or liver tissue at the first sign of GVH. Analyzing these specimens under the microscope provides a fairly accurate picture of any problems that might be arising, and permits us to initiate treatment with steroids and/or cyclosporine.

In early July, thirty-six days after entering the bone marrow transplant unit, Per went home to his family. At first, he needed to make frequent trips to a hematology clinic near his home for continued platelet transfusions and close examination for graft-versus-host disease. In late July, a rash appeared on his ears, palms, and forearms. He also had lost eight or nine pounds. We obtained a skin biopsy, which revealed a mild case of graft-versus-host disease. We treated his GVH with cyclosporine for several weeks, and were successful in arresting it before it caused serious damage.

Like acute GVH, chronic GVH can affect the skin, liver, and gastrointestinal tract. The chronic nature, however, leads to some unique problems, including dry, leathery skin, and hair loss due to the death of the hair follicles. In addition, persistent GVH in the intestine produces chronic diarrhea, poor absorption of food, and weight loss. Finally, people with chronic GVH have crippled immune systems. Their platelet count is low, so they may bleed; their white count is reduced, so they are susceptible to infection. Pulmonary disease may also arise. The treatment for chronic GVH is much like the immunosuppression employed in solid organ transplants—cyclosporine, azathioprine, and prednisone.

At Home

Because the immune system is still not fully reconstituted for a full six to twelve months after bone marrow transplantation, after going home recipients must take some special precautions to prevent infection. Even before the patient is discharged from the hospital, it is important to clean the house thoroughly, especially removing dust and molds from the draperies, carpets, and winter coats. During this vulnerable period, the recipient should wear a surgical mask when out in public, and should also avoid malls, busy shopping centers, and other crowded places where there is a high likelihood of being exposed to infectious agents. Particular care must be taken during the fall and spring flu seasons. Spread by little droplets from coughing and breathing, influenza viruses are extremely contagious and potentially life-threatening to anyone whose immune system is not entirely normal. In general, we suggest that recipients stay close to home for the first six months to a year. That means several months of refraining from working or attending concerts or large social gatherings. Above all, it is essential to avoid contact with anyone who may be even slightly ill.

> Twelve months after leaving the hospital, Per returned to work. Right now we are all expecting that he will be able to lead a normal life. Currently, he is off cyclosporine and other medications, and independent of transfusions. He has had no evidence of his cancer or further graft-versus-host disease. His bone marrow transplant appears to be a success.

The Hope of Bone Marrow Transplantation

While offering a potential cure for leukemia, lymphoma, bone cancer, and some relatively uncommon blood disorders, bone marrow transplantation is not for everyone. Although several scientific breakthroughs have occurred recently in the field, the procedure is still potentially dangerous, sometimes even fatal, and requires the coordinated expertise of many different medical specialists and supporting professionals. Many uses of bone marrow are still experimental, and hence not for general use outside of the university hospital or research institute. The enormous human resources, plus the special physical plant, needed to make BMT possible, are not now commonly found in most cities, and certainly exist in few, if any, community hospitals. This situation is not likely to change any time in the near future. The commitment by recipient and family also must span many months. Finally, not all states and insurance companies will cover the cost of the transplant, which in 1988 averaged from $100,000 to $150,000. Despite these words of caution, many people can benefit—potentially even be cured of an otherwise fatal illness—from bone marrow transplantation.

We expect that in the 1990s several developing technologies, such as hematologic growth factors, antiviral drugs, and safer chemotherapeutic agents, will work in concert to improve the success rate of bone marrow transplantation. As a result, we hope also to reduce the length of hospital stay and the cost. Critical to the overall success rate will be our ability to shorten the length of time when the poly count is low, thereby limiting the risk of serious infection. Another major breakthrough would be finding a way to completely control graft-versus-host disease in allogenic transplants. This would eliminate the need to find HLA matches and would make BMT widely available. This would, of course, require major advances in the field of immunology. However, while we wait for wider allogenic transplantation to become a reality, new names of potential bone marrow donors are being added to the computer registry. Perhaps by the year 2000 many—even most—Americans will have a potential unrelated donor on the list. Then, should one need BMT, a donor could be readily found. Finally, our hope is to expand bone marrow transplantation to the list of treatments for inherited diseases, such as sickle-cell anemia.

10

Living with a Transplant

This chapter is told in the words of the recipients and their loved ones participating in a heart transplant support group. It recounts their experiences going through the waiting, the surgery and recovery, going home, the setbacks, and the difficult, but rewarding, process of rehabilitation. Although they are heart recipients, we believe their thoughts and feelings will be helpful for anyone needing a transplant—regardless of the organ.

In addition to thanking everyone in the group for so willingly sharing their experiences and insights, we would like to give special thanks to Carol, who offered the diary she kept about her husband's heart transplant. As you read it—taking in her highs and lows—keep in mind that at this writing Carol is pregnant; enlarging their family shows the hope and faith she and Mike have in Mike's new heart. Their experience underscores the words of another member of the group: "Life is great, the second time around!"

Waiting

A man called me up who was waiting for a new heart. He said, "What happens if you don't make it?" I said, "You're gonna die. Look at it this way. If you don't have

it you're gonna die. And, if you do have it done, you
have a helluva chance to live." When I was waiting I
looked at those odds, and in my mind there was really
no choice there. "Have it done," I told him. He started to
ask, "What happens if . . . ?" I interrupted him: "Don't
even think about it. Just have it done."

$\bullet \quad \bullet \quad \bullet$

People call me and ask, "Should I have a transplant? My
doctor says I have to have one." I tell them point blank,
"I don't know, it's up to you." That was stressed on me
before the operation by my own doctor. He said to my
wife, "Don't try to talk him into it. He has to make up
his own mind."

$\bullet \quad \bullet \quad \bullet$

My doctor said to me, "In about ten years we'll think
about getting you a transplant." But by nine months later
I was having my transplant.

$\bullet \quad \bullet \quad \bullet$

Just keep on thinking, "There's a light at the end of the
tunnel." I was in the hospital for a month waiting for my
first operation. My doctor said, "If this doesn't work,
we'll send you to Pittsburgh for a new pump." I didn't
really know what he meant at the time, but he turned
out to be a prophet.

$\bullet \quad \bullet \quad \bullet$

The doctors want to know if you are ready to have it
done. If you go in with the wrong attitude, they don't
want to waste their time. They don't want to waste an
organ. You have to want to fight for everything after.

$\bullet \quad \bullet \quad \bullet$

I have to say that my faith has changed for the better.
I've gotten used to the fragility of life. At the end, before
the operation, I wasn't sure what the outcome would be
and worried, "I know I need this new heart, but will it be
there for me when I need it? When there is no more
time?" I developed trust and faith along the way. I guess

it was always there before my illness, but certainly not
quite as strong. I would pray, "You know, I really need
you now, God."

I remember just before the operation when my doctor
came in and said, "You're going downstairs in ten minutes." My mouth dropped. I said to myself, "I know this
is why I'm here, but am I really ready?" Then I thought,
"I am ready. I can't go on this way, and the sooner we
get on with it the better." My last thought was, "God,
I'm not sure what you have in mind for me. I know what
I have in mind for myself, but if they don't happen to be
the same, and things go another way . . . well, they say
you are merciful. So, let's go." So, when it really came
down to it, I had lost the fear. I had a feeling of serenity
to help me carry on. God gives you what you need when
you need it. I needed the courage and I got it. Now,
when I thank Him every day for being here, I also feel I
have the strength to handle whatever is next in line.

•   •   •

I drove back from the hospital in tears. The doctor had
said that there was no hope for him. "Look at his age,
his condition. There's nothing we can do for him." In the
hospital his heart was failing, his pressure was so low, he
was almost out of this world. But then a new heart became available. It saved his life. Now, when I look at
him, I can't believe it."

Transplant Diary

Wednesday, November 2, 5:30 A.M.
Dr. D. called, said we had a donor. Mary drove us to
Boston, arrived around 8:00 in the Emergency Room.
They prepped Mike. Heart from Newton. They took Mike
from ER at 1:30. Sally [transplant coordinator] came out
to sign papers, said heart was due at 2:30. Note came at
7:30, said operation was over, Mike moving to recovery.

Sally and Dr. D. came down, said things went pretty good. Had a problem with the medication to thicken his blood, had an allergic reaction. Tough going for a while, but should be no more problems. Went up to talk to Dr. V.—he did operation . . . Dr. D. wouldn't say how old donor was. Said there's a 15–20 percent chance might have some problem with bleeding, but heart looked very good. Got to see Mike for 10 minutes—looked good.

Thursday, November 3
Kept Mike sedated and paralyzed so he won't move and to give the heart's right side a chance to rest. Heart has a hard time getting used to the new body. Will start working on cutting down his meds to wake him up to get the respirator out. 9:30 P.M. visit: Mike was awake and recognized my voice—was doing good.

Friday, November 4
Mike was awake and waved to us when they took his respirator tube out at 11:30. Visit at 1:30, he could talk to us. He was very tired but would wake up for a visit. 5:30, Dr. D. said he's doing really good. Dr. V. will start taking out some of the stomach tubes Saturday and some Sunday. I might be able to get into the room. 7:30 visit, he was tired and was complaining of some pain in the chest. Gave a shot of morphine. At 9:30 visit he was really tired and still had a little discomfort. They started him on ice chips today. Complained at 1:30 he was getting hungry.

Saturday, November 5
Mike had a very tiring and emotional day. They took out 2 stomach tubes in the morning. Did a biopsy at 1:30. Dr. D. said his pressure and heart rate have been jumping around too much. It's either rejection or pericarditis—inflammation. Won't have results for 24 hours. Was eating supper at 7:30 visit—liquids. Got very emo-

tional on seeing everyone (Ma, Pat, Fred, and Dan).
Have to cut down on visitors.

Sunday, November 6
Still no word on biopsy. Had a little problem with his
heart rate jumping around. Gave him a shock treatment
to calm him down; try to get it under control. He was
resting good at 11:30, sleeping, peaceful. Heart rate and
blood pressure looked good. 1:30, Mike was sitting up
eating lunch. Did pretty good. 3:30, Betty and Ira came.
Mike was pretty alert and looked good. 5:30–7:30, was
pretty tired. 9:30, they had taken out one more of his
tubes. The catheter came out at 7:30. Hopefully, news
tomorrow on biopsy.

Monday, November 7
11:30 visit, Mike was sleeping. Laura, nurse, said he was
sitting and ate all his breakfast, so he was tired. 1:30, was
awake. Dr. V. stopped in. Biopsy negative. Finally got to
go in the room; felt so good to be near him emotions
flowed. 3:30, still doing good. Psychiatrist said he was
doing good. 5:30, got to stay for 1 hour 45 minutes to
feed him supper. He said Dr. D. and Sally stopped in,
said they would do another biopsy Thursday or Friday.
If goes well he'll be moved to another room, and if he
keeps going we'll be home for Thanksgiving.

Tuesday, November 8
Mike was good today. They pulled some of his pacer
wires, he's sore from that. Got up for a long time morning, afternoon, and night. Ate pretty well. Dr. D. said he
was doing good. Probably do a biopsy Monday. Kept the
pacer hooked cause heart rate was low (Kate nurse nice).
Charlie and Sue came to visit, handled it good. They also
took out his needle for blood gas. Right arm and legs

pretty swelled. Psychiatrist came again, said doing okay. Seems a little down cause he wants to do more but doesn't have the energy.

Wednesday, November 9
Mike did real good today. Sat up most of the morning and afternoon, ate real good. Still got emotional when he saw Ma. Dr. V. said they'll do a biopsy either Thursday, Friday, or Monday, but they might move him out Friday to upstairs. Feet and right arm still pretty swelled. Blood pressure has been good, heart rate usually high 70s low 80s. My first night home from Boston he seemed okay when I left. It felt so good to see Jeremy [their son]. Felt okay to be home, but we miss him so.

Thursday, November 10
Did another biopsy, should know Friday. Mike did very good eating and staying awake for being tired. Did biopsy because he's skipping beats.

Friday, November 11
Very tired today. The biopsy came back positive, shows some rejection. They put him on OKT3 to kill the white blood cells that are going after the heart. Also put him on a new pill for his skipped beats. Said medication working good. Will keep Mike in intensive care for the weekend and move him during the week if everything looks good.

Saturday, November 12
Mike was sick overnight. Very tired and stressed all day. He started to run a fever late afternoon. Dr. D. says its because of the OKT3. It will take a couple of days for his body to get used to it. His white blood count is low, so it's taking effect.

Sunday, November 13
Mike looked really good today. Said the doctor said he
was doing good, if everything goes good he can go upstairs Monday. Mike had a strange night, said he was
having bad dreams (hallucinations). The nurse was really
nice and sat with him until he felt better. He says it was
like his body was telling the OKT3 to go away. Bob, Pat,
Midas, Chris, Rene, and his wife came to say hi after the
meeting. Bob told us he was transplanted on the same
day. Charlie stopped by.

Monday, November 14
Mike was real good today. Still in intensive care. Dr. V.
wants him to stay because of irregular heartbeat. Maybe
Tuesday can move. They took another echocardiogram.
Mike was feeling bored by the end of the day. Anxious to
get out.

Tuesday, November 15
Mike had a bad mental day. He kept thinking he was
dead or dying, couldn't figure out what to say to stay
alive. Needed to say the Apostles' Creed. We (Mike, me,
and Mary Jane) tried to figure out the saying. When he
said Amen he broke down crying. After he calmed down
for a few minutes he wanted to finish washing up. They
moved him to the other floor at 4:00. He had trouble
from 11:30–3:00. He was still shaky and nervous about
what happened all night. Couldn't seem to relax. Dr. S.
(psychiatrist) thinks between the medication, the being
confined for so long, and not getting good nights of sleep
caused his problem.

Wednesday, November 16
Two weeks today. Mike was kinda blah today. Didn't talk
much. Said he remembered parts of yesterday. Didn't
really seem to want to talk so I didn't push it. Was very
shaky. Dr. said probably from the cyclosporine. He had a

problem with his tongue. Said it felt swollen. Dr. took a look at it. Didn't say much. Started with a fever late afternoon. They upped his OKT3. Thinks that's what's making the fever and he was skipping beats probably from the fever.

Thursday, November 17
Mike was better today. Still a little bored. He took a little walk to the end of the hall. Sat for a while and walked back. He was a little tired. Said Dr. D. said he needed six more days of OKT3. Next Wednesday, Thursday is Thanksgiving. Friday they're doing a biopsy and go from there.

Friday, November 18
Mike was real good today. Rode his bike for 7 minutes and walked to the echo lab. Tired him out pretty good. Charlie and John came to visit. Phil, Ricky, and Joe C. called last night. Goofy called today. Dr. D. says maybe Tuesday for the biopsy. Everything looks good so far.

Saturday and Sunday, November 19 and 20
Pat came up to visit with me. Mike was pretty good. Went for a walk down to the end of the hall and back. Tried to take a nap in the afternoon, couldn't get comfortable. Sunday was very good. Said he could focus and concentrate better. Phil, Goofy, and Billy came to visit. Was nice to see everyone. Bob also stopped by.

Monday, November 21
Janice came with me to visit. Mike was kind of tired. Said he'd been up at 4:30. Hadn't had any nap. His sugar was 39 [low] because he had a liquid lunch. Was supposed to have a biopsy at 3:00, rescheduled to 5:00, then they had an emergency and said they wouldn't be able to do him. Dr. D. said he wanted him done today. Finally took him at 7:15. Called him at 9:15 when I got home. Said was

finished by 8:30. Felt pretty good, not too tired. Had supper. Joey and Joyce were there visiting.

Tuesday, November 22
Mike had a really good day. Said he rode the bike two times for 5 minutes and walked the hall three times with the nurses. Said he felt really good. Sally came in and talked about what to do when he comes home. No driving for six weeks. No crowds for two weeks. Watch diet and let them know of any changes. Dr. D. came and said the biopsy looked good. The OKT3 was working. The rejection is subsiding. Hopefully the skip beats will go when the rejection goes. The echo showed some fluid build-up around the heart. They can take that out with a needle. Outlook good, stay on OKT3 through weekend. Another biopsy next week. If everything looks good, shooting for the weekend [for discharge].

Wednesday, November 23
Mike had the fluid drained. Said it hurt bad. They got him nervous because they called Dr. D. and Dr. V. Dr. D. said it was because the fluid was orange instead of yellow. But it doesn't seem anything is up with it. Dr. D. said hopefully next Thursday [for discharge].

Thursday, November 24 (Thanksgiving)
Mike said Dr. V. said he wasn't sure how much longer on the OKT3. Maybe another 10 days. Drained his fluid some more. Said has to be off the OKT3 for 3 days before biopsy. We had a nice dinner. Mike was pretty tired most of the day. Couldn't seem to get comfortable to nap.

Friday, November 25
Mike was pretty good today. A little tired. Dr. V. drained more fluid. Pretty sure they stopped the OKT3 today. Made 14 days. Someone mentioned 18 but don't think they go that long. Dr. S.—cardiology—is going to start

him on a new medication for the arrhythmia. They're not sure what's causing it, so they want to try and stop it, or control it before it becomes a problem.

Saturday and Sunday, November 26 and 27
Mike did good all weekend. Still has some trouble with napping, but still feels good. Felt a flutter Sunday afternoon. They upped his Quinaglute and took out his catheter. Said that might be causing some of the problem. Big test: cardiac catheterization and biopsy Monday morning.

Monday, November 28
Mike had a busy day. They did a lot of tests—biopsy, cath, took pictures. Took 3 hours. He was real tired. Dr. D. said the pictures looked good. The heart sounds and is working good. He had to keep the sand bag on until 8 P.M. and stay in bed until morning. Echo in the morning.

Tuesday, November 29
Mike was a lot better today. Rode his bike twice for 7 minutes. We walked the hall 4 times up and back. He did real good. No shortness of breath. Said he took his first shower today. Felt like a new man. Dr. D. came in around 5:00. No results yet. Will call us. Called around 6:30—good report—no rejection—the echo looked good. A little fluid, but not too bad—will probably watch him for a day or two for the arrhythmia and get last-minute details. Probably come home Friday morning.

Wednesday, November 30
Mike did real good today. Rode the bike for 7 minutes and 15 minutes. Walked twice up and down the hallway. Dr. D. said they want to do a stress test. So it'll be either Friday morning or afternoon.

Thursday, December 1

Mike did his stress test today. Didn't do good. Had some ectopies [irregular beats]. Dr. D. says he'll have to stay until it's settled down. They started him on a new medication and told him to do as much as he can this weekend. They'll do another stress test Monday. I got home and Billy and Goofy were scraping the walls. They put the bed back together and found a note in back of the bed. It was a letter from Mike telling everyone how he felt and loved them. A letter in case anything happened to him.

Friday, December 2

Mike put up the tension on his bike. Rode it twice. He seemed tired and like something was bothering him. But he said he felt all right. Dr. D. stopped in. Said they were on for Monday stress test. Told them to start off slow and work him up and they would do an echo, too. I told Mike about finding the letter. He said I was supposed to find it. Just wanted to let me know how he felt just in case. I told him to start talking to me more or write it down, so I can help instead of being left out.

Saturday, December 3

Mike was tired today. Feet pretty puffy. Dr. V. told him to keep them up. He did ride the bike and went for a walk 2 times up and back. Tried to catch up on his rest.

Sunday, December 4

Mike finally got to see Jeremy today. Jeremy was a little hesitant with the mask, but it went pretty well. Mike was so glad to see him. Dr. D. told Mike Monday the stress test and echo. Tuesday a biopsy. If the echo shows fluid they have to drain it out. Probably 2 days for the catheter to drain. If the stress test goes good, yeah! If not, more different medications. If biopsy good, discharge probably end of the week.

Monday, December 5
Caught Mike in the elevator going upstairs. Said it went well. The guy told him last time he had lots of palpitations and ectopies in a row. This time no palpitations and 2 ectopies. He called and Dr. D. was pleased. Dr. D. was gone for the night so we did not get his full report on the stress test and echo. Mike felt that everything went real good.

Recovering

I think the minute I woke up I felt wonderful. I'm certain that I looked like a horror show, but I knew that physically everything was better. It must have been the circulation. I couldn't verbalize it, the breathing tube was in my throat. But I remember asking for a piece of paper and a pencil, so I could write down my first thoughts. My initial reaction was, "I made it. I feel better." I looked down and saw the mess of a chest that I had—it was all covered up in bandages, of course—but I still didn't care.

•   •   •

I remember in intensive care, seeing him there with all the tubes and the bandages. I said, "Oh my God, his hair's changed!" It looked darker, healthier. He had light hair before the operation and then it turned dark brown. Maybe it was the circulation. But oh how I thanked God he was alive.

•   •   •

On waking up, one of the first things I remember is that I couldn't feel my heart. I had had years of pain, and irregular heart rhythms. I was always unsure of my heart. Normal people don't think about their heart. It just beats. When I woke up from surgery I remember think-

ing, "I can't feel my heart. I'm better!" And I still feel
that way. It's just a normal heart pumping away.

•   •   •

The surgeon came in and said, "You're having massive
rejection and we don't know what to do with you. We're
having a meeting to discuss it." I looked at my husband
and he broke down. That was the first time he cried, he
thought he was going to die.

I went out of the room to find the surgeon. I was on
the verge of breaking down, too, but I didn't want to cry
in front of my husband. I was terrified. I found the doctor down the hall. He was in with another patient, so I
waited until he came out of the room. "What do you
mean?" I asked, and started crying. It was the first time I
had broken down. It was the uncertainty, the fear.

Another doctor came and said, "Let's go to the cafete-
ria." When we got there he said, "We'll fix it. I'm sorry
about the way it came off. It's hard to deal with bad
news and some of us have more difficulty than others.
We'll change the medications. Hang in. Don't lose hope.
We'll try OKT3"—which at that point was an experimental medication. "If that doesn't work, we'll try another
heart." When it was all over, we went out to dinner. My
husband broke his diet a bit, and had fettuccine Alfredo,
perhaps in jest, but also in honor of his doctor, whose
first name is Alfred.

•   •   •

After the operation I started thinking, "Well I needed a
new part and now I have it, so let's get on with it." By
that I meant, "I have the new heart so it's time to start
living again"—physically, psychologically. A lot has to do
with the psychological, and everyone has to do it their
own way. But the emotional part was something they
had not done a whole lot with in the hospital where I
had my operation. They hadn't addressed it, so I had to
find my own way of dealing with it. At first, there were
days when I couldn't even get my legs moving, because

the muscles were gone. But I wasn't going to take that
sitting down, either literally or figuratively. "Great,
you've got a new heart, but your legs don't work." So,
each day, I would push out of that chair. Some days I
would push, but still not be able to get up.

Pretty soon everything was moving. A little slow, but
moving. I felt that with time, and patience, everything
would be a bit better.

•   •   •

Someone I respect said to me, "You don't have a heart
problem any more." I was taken aback. It's very hard to
envision, but my heart problem had become part of me. I
had a hard time accepting that the old problem was
gone. I had that problem for seven years. I don't expect it
will take me seven years to feel like I don't have a heart
problem any more, but it won't come overnight either.

Coming Home

I felt very safe in the hospital, because the entire staff
was there. Every time I had a little ache or pain, I'd press
the button and someone would come to calm me. Even if
it was nothing it was still a security blanket kind of thing.
The very first night being away from the hospital, we still
weren't home. I had the operation in Pittsburgh, and we
had to stay over in the apartment we were renting. I was
happy to be out of the hospital, but I still couldn't sleep
one second. I was a little leery. "What if something happens?" I worried. "What will I do now?" I knew what
medications to take, the proper amount, and when to
take them, because I'd been going over that for weeks
before leaving. I knew the exercise routine I was supposed to go through. Everything was in my head and
written down. But I still had the fear of this thing they
gave me—the new heart. I used to put my hand on my
chest to see if it felt different from my own heart. I
couldn't tell the difference from the way my own heart

felt when it was healthy. But until I was on the plane coming home I still didn't feel right. And when we got home I asked my wife to take off the sheets that had been on the bed before the operation—when my heart was failing. It was crazy, but I just felt that I couldn't sleep on them.

●   ●   ●

I was home alone for a while after Betty went back to work. She would call me up and ask, "Are you okay?" My friends would also call every hour, to make sure I was okay. It took a month for all of us to calm down.

●   ●   ●

After I came back from the hospital, my wife stayed home with me for about two weeks. Then she went back to work and I felt like I was on a solo flight for the first time—alone, in the cockpit, flying the plane. Before my operation I had had a lifeline hookup around my neck. You know, press a button and the ambulances come. All that was stripped, now. I didn't need that. But what if something happened?

●   ●   ●

When he was leaving the hospital, I asked the doctors, "How long should he recuperate?" They said, "Not a minute. He's got a new heart. He should use it, as long as it lasts." The message was, "Don't walk on eggshells. You don't have to live in a cocoon. Put it in first, and let it rip."

●   ●   ●

Being young, I said to myself, "Jeez, when I get transplanted I'm going to be out of the hospital in ten days." I wanted to set a world record. Then you get done, and you feel, "This isn't so easy. I'm going to be here a little longer."

Now I reflect back and give other people a lot of credit. It's a struggle and I'm only thirty years old. It's hard to get on the bike and pedal every day, to motivate yourself. Everybody expects that you'll be right back on your feet, since you waited so long for the operation. It took six years for me to deal with getting sick, and having the operation. I'm slowly, but surely, getting my strength back. And my confidence is coming back, too. Psychologically, you can't say, "I don't feel right today. I'm just going to lie in bed all day." You have to say, "It's just a bad day," and get yourself going.

• • •

I know I'm going to have some bad days. I remind myself that I've had days like this before, and that tomorrow will probably be better. The next day I'll be able to get out and go for a walk. People ask, "How're you doing?" and I think they want me to say "Fine," even if I don't feel so fine.

• • •

The hardest part is when you try to do something that bogs everyone else down. You know, taking a walk and feeling everyone has to wait for me. Before my operation I was always fifteen feet behind my wife. I spent a couple of years saying, "I'm comin', I'm comin', it's okay." And she was doing the grocery shopping and carrying the bags. Your family doesn't complain, your friends don't complain, but it preys on your mind. You still feel it.

• • •

At first, I found it hard to accept John being at home. Every time he breathed the wrong way, I'd be ready to call the ambulance. I really had a bad time of it. For a long time I felt like I was sleeping with my eyes open. The doctor said, "You may never get over this feeling, but you should remember that if there's a complication, it's not going to be sudden. He's not going to go fast." I had a hard time accepting that he was okay now. When I was coming home from work, if I saw an ambulance anywhere near the house, I would panic. I was used to jumping at every little sound or motion. It still happens and it's five years later. Sometimes he gets up at night with a cramp in his legs. I wake up too, and I'm worried.

Day to Day

The other day, we were at a party for the new officers of
our club. He was walking around in his tuxedo. People's
eyes were watering, he looked so good. His mother came
over. Her eyes were watering, too. She said, "I couldn't
stand it, seeing him walk around, knowing what it had
been like before, not walking from here to there. Now,
he's so sure of himself." Then he came over and I gave
him a big kiss. "You look great," I said. He looked at me
and said, "I'm so happy to just be able to walk and talk.
It's been a year and a half since the transplant. Time just
seems to have zoomed by. It seems like it was yesterday
that I was going into the operating room."

       •   •   •

Being a cardiac patient for so long—over twenty years—I
knew that the worst thing is to cripple yourself afterward
by not doing things after surgery. So many people don't
do as much as they can. You really gotta push yourself.
Once you do something once, you won't be so afraid to
do it again. It seems like so many people hold themselves
back when they don't need to. After the surgery, I had
some apprehension the first time I went skiing. Now, I
go skiing alone. I go deep in the woods cross-country
skiing. I don't feel in any more danger than anyone else.

When I was a kid, I saw that the parents often held
back other kids who had heart disease. They were told
not to let them do things. Now they tell them, "Let 'em
go." It's up to your support group—your family and
friends—not to hold you back. My mother has been great
with that over the years. When they were telling her to
hold me back from doing things, she was great. She
knew I wouldn't be happy living like that. I would go off
hiking in the woods, because that's what I love to do.
She didn't know how long I would live, but she knew it
wouldn't be fair for me not to be able to do those things.
I've been told by my doctors that I would have died a

long time ago if I hadn't done the things that I did. There were times when I just barely made it, but got through because my lungs were strong. Well, that's because I did the hiking, and because my will is strong.

· · ·

Jim had his transplant more than five years ago. He plays softball, even though he says he sometimes has cramps in his legs. He was just over forty when he had the operation, so now he's in his late forties. That's pretty good for anyone his age. I can remember watching his family go through the operation and the time after, and wondering, "How can a family go through all that?" Little did we know that a year later we would be going through the same thing.

· · ·

The other morning I went out and my neighbor said, "How're you doing?" I said, "Good, good." He said, "I was talking to somebody about a month ago who said you weren't doing good at all." I laughed. "Tell me about it," I said to him as a joke. "That's news to me. But you should have come by yourself to find out."

· · ·

I always had a hard time in school, but the memory problem has affected that. Right now I'm taking all art courses, mostly labs where I'm in the darkroom working on my photography. So it doesn't really bother me. I'm going to be starting academics again, so I'll have to deal with it. I definitely have a short-term-memory loss. Getting back to school was great. It was wonderful to be real busy. The worst thing is not having anything to do. I'm going to an art school, so it's a whole lot of fun to be able to work at something you enjoy. Practically no one I go to school with knew I had a heart transplant. And people I know outside of school didn't really relate to me differently, because I'd been a heart patient practically all of my life. This was just another phase, not a shock for anyone.

My friends look at me and say, "You're the closest thing to a miracle I've ever personally encountered." The ones who knew me when I was really sick now see me after the transplant and cannot believe it's the same person. I met a guy yesterday who said, "I heard something yesterday that I just cannot believe. You have a new heart." I said, "Yup." He said, "You don't look sick." I said, "Jeez, well I'm not. I'm well. You should have seen me a year and a half ago. I was sick then, but I'm well now. I'm as well as the next guy. At least, that's the way I feel." He just couldn't believe it.

• • •

Do you ever get to the point where you ask yourself, "From zero percent to 100 percent, where am I now?" After six months, after a year. I remember someone asking me, "How long did it take before you started feeling good?" One guy said it took him about two years before he was feeling 100 percent. I don't mean getting out and running, but how you feel personally, inside. I feel better now than before I had my major coronary. I was overweight, I never did any exercise. I was too busy to enjoy life. All of a sudden, bang. My heart went. And then I learned to stop to smell the flowers. It's not going to happen like that again. I work, but it's different. I get up in the morning and say, "Thank you, Lord." I take it one day at a time. I've stopped saying to myself, "I've gotta do this, I've gotta plan for that." I'd never go back to the rat race.

• • •

There was a time when I thought, "I'll never be able to lift up my grandson, or see Joanne or Bob." I figured there were all the things I wanted to see, that I would never get a chance to see. I had tears in my eyes when my grandson came to visit me in the hospital before the transplant. He was just a little baby and I couldn't pick him up. It drove me crazy. I cried so hard when no one was around. How could I not hold him, and hug him, and pick him up? Now, that's all different. It feels great. Those are things you dream about, and I was being deprived of that. But not any more.

. . .

We have another one on the way! I never thought I'd be able to say that. Months ago I remember driving back from the movies with my son on my lap. I was hugging him and thinking to myself, "This is the first time I've been able to hug him like this—ever!" I got sick just before he was born. He's three now, and I had never been able to pick him up and hug him. Tears came to my eyes. I could be like any other father.

. . .

I'm planning a trip to Venezuela. I plan on staying with friends down there who have a home. I know it will be very clean. I'd be somewhat afraid to drink the public water, or eat whatever might be considered fast food, but otherwise I'm looking forward to it. I asked my doctor about any shots that might be necessary. And we talked about general precautions. His suggestions were basically good commonsense ideas. Nothing very special. I'm very excited about the trip.

. . .

It used to be that we were supposed to wear masks when we went out. For instance, five years ago when I left the hospital for the first time after the transplant, we asked about a restaurant in town. We wanted to celebrate, but didn't know where to eat. My doctor suggested what was probably the most popular restaurant in town. This restaurant was crowded—very crowded—and we had to wait in line right next to other people. I didn't feel like wearing a mask. It made me feel self-conscious. Finally, we were seated. The first course came and I was ravenous. You know, we would have eaten anything after the hospital food. But, anyway, the woman next to me at another table takes in a big breath and sneezes all over my face. I'm looking at my wife and she's in panicsville. I told my doctor that I hadn't been wearing the mask. How can you eat with a mask on anyway? He said, "Aw, don't worry about it. We don't know if it works anyway."

. . .

I was scared at first. Don't do this, don't do that. But what are you going to do, stay in the house all the time?

. . .

To get to my school, I have to ride the subway all the time. So, I'm exposed to stuff all the time. I try to eat well, get plenty of rest and exercise, and just live my life. So far this winter I've been healthier than anyone else in my class.

. . .

I got out of the hospital in January. By that April we were in Florida. One couple was from there, so we stayed with them. I was nervous making the reservations because we couldn't cancel them. "What if I get sick?" I thought. "We'd lose that money."

. . .

We did the same thing. I got out of the hospital at the very end of November and by the first of February we were in Florida. The doctors said that it was okay to travel, and that we should check in with a nearby hospital. So we called ahead to a hospital in West Palm Beach, made arrangements to have some blood work done while we were there, and everything was fine. We found out what we should do if we had an emergency. The hospital assured us that there was nothing to worry about. I don't know about a cruise. Being in the middle of the ocean and having something happen would make me nervous, even though I know that it's unlikely that something will happen quickly. But the cruise would still make me a little nervous. Otherwise traveling has been great. This year we spent five weeks in Florida.

· · ·

I check my blood pressure every day. At first, I took it twice a day. Now I take it first thing in the morning before I get out of bed. I have a cuff right next to my bed. I just about haven't missed a day.

· · ·

I take my pressure about three times a week. When I first got out, I used to take it every day.

· · ·

I don't take my blood pressure at all, only when I go for my regular medical visits.

Exercising

I was back at school two months after my transplant and skiing four months afterward. I walk about an hour a day. I walk a lot on my way to school and back. I feel better than I ever have my whole life. I don't worry about the skiing. I take any trail I can handle.

· · ·

Two weeks after my surgery, I was on a stationary bike in the hospital. After discharge I went through a physical therapy program at a nearby hospital. I went a few days a week and was able to get my heart rate up on the stationary bicycle, eventually up to about 125–128 [beats a minute] without any problem. My legs gave out first, even before my breathing. The first ten minutes I'd hit the wall and then get through it. My legs would start calming down and I would get going again. Now that the weather is better I'm walking regularly. I try to do a mile or two a day.

· · ·

I exercise three times a week in a cardiac rehab program at a hospital. I work out on the bicycle, treadmill, rowing machine, stairmaster, and weights. I really need it. It

keeps my blood pressure down, and my energy up.
When I wasn't doing the workout I'd fall asleep on the
couch after dinner. Now I've got a lot more energy. I
could use the bike at home too. It's not that I'm afraid to
exercise on my own, it's just that I won't do it unless I go
somewhere and have other people to urge me on. If I
don't show up for a couple of days, people get on my
case. "Where the heck were you?" they kid me. But it
never entered my head that I might be alone exercising
and something would happen. It's just my motivation. I
do sometimes pick up the weights at home. I don't worry
about passing out or anything.

                    •   •   •

I don't do any exercise. When I get worked up my heart
races and I have to take a beta blocker. When I take my
stress test I have fast runs and palpitations. Then, at
eight months after, I was on two pills for the arrhythmia.
After a while on the beta blocker I was scheduled for the
stress test. I got all wired up, and saw the fella get the
paddles ready, just in case something happened to my
heart rhythm. Jeez, I got scared. "No way," I said. I think
its just the fear factor. I don't want to be a world athlete.
I just want to see my wife, the baby, and enjoy life a little
bit.

     My doctor said, "What if your son is in the pool and
he's drowning, and you have to go in after him? Could
you handle it?" I had never thought of it like that. I don't
know to this day if I could run up to the next building.
I'm afraid to try. I think I should be exercising, but I'm
not.

                    •   •   •

I don't exercise, but I feel I have a lot of energy. I'm up
at six with the baby, and in bed after eleven.

                    •   •   •

I used to be a good bowler, but now I can't control the
ball. Maybe the boy whose heart I have wasn't a good
bowler. It makes me aggravated when the ball goes down

the gutter. I have the mechanics, but I can't get the ball down the middle. It's the rhythm. Can't seem to do it. And then I said, "What am I getting aggravated about? Do something else." That was it for the bowling.

• • •

After I was discharged I used to walk to a nearby hospital for a rehab program. I specifically went up a steep hill. After the exercise routine I would walk back, too. That lasted about four months, and I started losing the discipline. It was mental, even though the exercise felt great. I don't know what it was that I stopped and I lost the discipline. There was no one there to kick my butt and say get out there.

• • •

A problem for me was that before the transplant I had spent three or four years of doing nothing. You know, the doctors had said, "Don't lift, don't strain." And I had been in bed a lot. So I wasn't used to getting out there and exercising. For a while after the transplant, I said to myself, "You've gotta get out there and get moving." But soon I was back to my old self.

• • •

Every night I go to the supermarket. That's my job, I do the shopping. But I always leave out something from the list, so I have to go back the next day. I do that because in the supermarket I make sure to walk all the aisles. I take the carriage and go through the whole store, sometimes a couple of times. A lot of times it's cold or raining outside, or even too hot. The supermarket is temperature-controlled.

Working

I started back working three mornings a week, nine to one. I look forward to going to work. I find it very relaxing, and it gives me a feeling of being back in the mainstream. It's not a question of getting rich, but more like not being in the routine of having no purpose. It gets me dressed, shaved, I put on the shirt and tie. I meet people. I appreciate the days off more. I don't think I could handle nine to five, five days a week. I think there would be more stress.

Loved Ones and Other Supports

It's easy to forget how rough it is on the partner. Everyone's always saying, "How's the patient, how's the patient?" But you're dragging. You haven't slept in a year and a half. But when they ask you, "How do you feel?" you say, "Oh, fine," but you don't feel that way.

·   ·   ·

People that you never suspect will help, they send a card or a donation. We had a party for Pete over at the Elks, three floors, three bands. It was awesome. Everyone donated their time.

·   ·   ·

It's scary watching others in the hospital. There was a room for talking to the families. They brought in another family and told them some bad news. Doctors and nurses learn from the "Deadpan School." You don't know what's going on behind their eyes. When the doctor came in, he said I could go in to see my husband in about an hour. That was at 10:30. Well, 11:30 went by, 12:30 went by, and 1:30 went by. I'm sitting there and I was a wreck. The nurse came in and said, "I'm sorry. He woke up and we had an awful job cleaning him up." For her it wasn't much, but I was terrified the whole time.

·   ·   ·

When I was wheeled off to the operating room my wife said, "Wait a minute, there's something more I want to say." She was thinking, "What if something happens and he doesn't come back?" There would always be something more we both wanted to say. The doctor's attitude was, "Let's get on with it." I suppose he knew it was going to turn out okay. For him, it was like an appendix operation. My final words were, "See ya later." I think that's why I made it through (chuckle). I told her I was going to see her later, so it was a promise. When I woke up, I wrote two things down on a piece of paper—I had the respirator still in: "What time is it?" and "Where's my wife?" I'd made that promise. I don't know why I cared about the time, because I promptly forgot it. But I didn't forget the promise to my wife.

• • •

The people around you help a lot by keeping you positive. There's a lot of stuff that you have to deal with afterward. They make a big difference.

• • •

I got a call, yesterday, from Jeff's sister. She said that he's been having a rough time. He and Betty broke up. She said his mental state was very bad. Before the transplant, his wife was in total charge. After the transplant he wanted to take over, and she didn't like the idea. I'm sure there's a lot more to it than that. I guess she couldn't handle the whole situation. It seems so strange that they could stay together waiting, and then break up after the worst part of the ordeal is over. You need all the support after, trying to get back in the mainstream. You've been walking on eggshells so long. Waiting and waiting.

• • •

One of the things I wondered when I first came home was, "How fast will I get back on my feet?" My doctor said, "You're doing just fine at this stage." I'd say back, "Fine, but as opposed to who?" No answer. You know, if I had had a bypass I could go two streets in any direction and talk to someone who'd had that operation. And even though my doctor would often say, "Don't worry about it," I usually wanted to talk with someone I could compare notes with. But who could I talk to who had a transplant? My doctor's response was, "I don't know of

anyone." There was a local Heart Association group, but
that's for people with heart problems. I don't have a
heart problem. My heart is new. My problems have to do
with a suppressed immune system. So we started a heart
transplant association.

.   .   .

It's hard to go through it. But you know your loved one
won't be there without it. He didn't have a future to begin with, so you take the chance.

.   .   .

I had my operation at another hospital. The physical part
of the operation wasn't bad, but my doctors didn't address the psychological aspects at all. I had to find my
own way. They relied on patients' helping patients. We
really didn't know what to expect. I said to Beth that if
something goes wrong, and they have to go in again, I
would be a lot less scared. I'd know what I'd be going
through. I'd know there would be happy days, but also
days when I couldn't seem to wake up.

.   .   .

For me, there was no choice in having it done. But the
support group took a load off my mind. Going to the
group before made me feel a lot more at ease.

.   .   .

We sell bumper stickers, sweatshirts, send a letter to
every cardiologist in the state to let them know we're
here. We don't charge anything. We don't proselytize.
It's all strictly voluntary. All of us are in it to help others,
but it does an awful lot for me. I get back more than I
give when I talk to others. I'm in seventh heaven. It
makes me feel like I'm giving something back for everything I've gotten. And we're all in this thing together.
Being there for someone else. I don't care how long
you've been out. There are times when you need to pick

up the phone and talk about what's bothering you. Large things, small things, even trivial ones.

Thinking about the Donor

About a week after the operation I realized that I was having some psychological problems. I found that I was, all the time, still thanking anyone who had anything to do with the surgery—thanking them up and down and in every direction. I was so grateful for the second chance. "What is it I'm groping for?" I asked myself. After much thought it came to me. I had not been able to thank the people who had been responsible for my being here. I had thanked God, the doctors, the nurses, but here it finally came to me. "I haven't been able to say thank-you to the people who had given me my new heart."

Realizing that it is an anonymous program, I still felt that need to say thank-you. I said to the surgeon, "I'm having just one problem. If I write a letter, will you see that it goes where I want it to go?" He proceeded to tell me just a little about the person from whom I received my organ. It was a twenty-year-old girl who was in the process of having a baby when she died. And so I said a prayer for her and her family.

I realize what a big decision that is. When you lose someone you care about, and at that point someone is asking you to donate the person's organs. Wow! And to say, "Yes, I'll do that," takes a lot. I can relate to that because I lost a daughter in her first year of life. But it happened very quickly and no one asked me to donate. I'm looking back, and had I been asked, it would have been a complete shock. I might have said, "Do you know what you are asking?" Maybe then it would have been totally inconceivable that someone would have approached me with that question. But now I know what it means, and I wrote it to the donor's family. Once I wrote that letter I felt a great release.

Complications

We take precautions against infection. Sometimes it feels like "Avoid, avoid, avoid." I've had a cold this week, so he's been sleeping on the third floor. He just stays away, as much as he can. It's very difficult around the house. I try to keep him away from hugging people, but everyone wants to hug him anyway. I tell him that he should extend his hand and keep them at arm's length.

•   •   •

I don't do that, even though I know my immune system is down compared to other people.

•   •   •

I've had fewer colds in the last year than ever in my life. I don't take Bactrim.

•   •   •

I take the Bactrim one week a month. I start about the 20th of the month and take two tablets a day for about a week. I don't take anything like Actifeds or Pseudofeds. I work in the garden in the summertime. I wear gloves sometimes, but not always, when I work in the garden.

•   •   •

I'm getting awful nervous. It seems like everyone I hear about is coming in with hepatitis. I have a biopsy coming up and I'm really scared about it. Non-A, non-B. I was in a few days with a colon infection. I worry that I'm going to get the hepatitis, too. I don't know where they're getting it from. Bill has it. Jennifer has it. It's usually transmitted through the blood. I had non-A, non-B in 1978 with my first bypass. I'm going to ask my doctor when I'm in for the biopsy. I'm not trying to scare anybody, but I want to know why it's happening all of a sudden.

•   •   •

I have some warts on my fingers. I've been having them treated, but they're stubborn. I figure the trade-off is well worth it. As long as my heart works. Periodically, I get some shakes. They say it's the medication. At first, it was brutal. I couldn't write my name. I felt embarrassed and frustrated. I'd put some peas on a fork and by the time it got up to my mouth there was nothing on it. There was one time, when I went to the hospital, that I couldn't even sign the release form. The girl said, "Don't worry about it, just sign it. Write your name, we know it's you." It was a month before I could write, but it went away. And I had some problems with memory. There was a time that I couldn't remember my Social Security number and even the Lord's Prayer. The Lord's Prayer is second nature. That was when I was in the hospital and when I first came home. But that went away, too, in a few weeks. Even now there are times when I have some short-term-memory loss.

Is It Worth It?

When people who are waiting for a transplant ask me, "Is it worth it?" I say, "Wow, hang in there, you're going to do it. It's wonderful afterward. I'd like to do it all over again, just to go through feeling so much better."

Acknowledgments

We would like to thank members of the MGH Heart Transplant Support Group, including George Bouret, Michael and Carol Weldon, Bob and Pat Jellison, Joan and David Barnes, Sister Agnes Buckley, Robert and Mary Coleman, Chris and Cecile Darcey, Tom and Louise Whelton, Louise and Al Leandro, and Claire Sylvia. We would also like to thank Camille Smith for her superb editorial comments.

Contributors

Hugh Auchincloss, Jr., M.D.
Associate Professor of Surgery, Harvard Medical School
Chief, Pancreatic Transplantation, MGH
Transplant Specialties: Liver, kidney, and pancreas transplantation

A. Benedict Cosimi, M.D.
Professor of Surgery, Harvard Medical School
Chief, Transplantation Service, MGH
Transplant Specialties: Liver, kidney, and pancreas transplantation

G. William Dec, M.D.
Assistant Professor of Medicine, Harvard Medical School
Medical Director, MGH Cardiac Transplantation Program
Transplant Specialties: Heart and heart-lung transplantation

Francis L. Delmonico, M.D.
Associate Professor of Surgery, Harvard Medical School
Director, Renal Transplantation, MGH
Transplant Specialties: Liver, kidney, and pancreas transplantation

Susan B. Grainger, R.N., M.S.
Head Nurse, Transplant Unit, MGH
Transplant Specialties: Liver, kidney, pancreas, heart, and lung
transplantation

John T. Herrin, M.B.B.S., F.R.A.C.P.
Associate Clinical Professor of Pediatrics, Harvard Medical School
Chief of Pediatric Nephrology and Pediatrician, MGH
Transplant Specialty: Pediatric kidney transplantation

Sally A. Keck, R.N.
Coordinator for Cardiac Surgery Patient Education, Cardiac Transplant
Coordinator, MGH
Transplant Specialty: Heart transplantation

H. F. Pizer
Medical writer and author of ten books about health and medicine

Robert H. Rubin, M.D.
Associate Professor of Medicine, Harvard Medical School
Chief, Infectious Disease for Transplantation, and Director, Clinical
Investigation Program, MGH
Transplant Specialty: Infection in the compromised host

Paul S. Russell, M.D.
John Homans Professor of Surgery, Harvard Medical School
Former Chief, Transplantation Unit, MGH

Michael Seiden, M.D.
Medical Chief Resident, MGH
Transplant Specialty: Bone marrow transplantation

Owen S. Surman, M.D.
Assistant Professor of Psychiatry, Harvard Medical School
Psychiatric Consultant, MGH Transplantation Unit
Transplant Specialties: Kidney, liver, pancreas, lung and heart
transplantation

Nina E. Tolkoff-Rubin, M.D.
Director, Hemodialysis and Continuous Ambulatory Peritoneal Dialysis
Units, and Medical Coordinator for the Renal Transplant Program, MGH
Associate Professor of Medicine, Harvard Medical School
Transplant Specialties: Kidney and pancreas transplantation

Gus J. Vlahakes, M.D.
Assistant Professor of Surgery, Harvard Medical School
Surgical Director, MGH Transplantation Program
Transplant Specialties: Heart and heart-lung transplantation

John C. Wain, M.D.
Instructor in Surgery, Harvard Medical School
Director, MGH Lung Transplantation Program
Transplant Specialty: Lung transplantation

Index